TESTIMONIALS

"I have enjoyed working with Geraldine throughout the years. The expertise and knowledge she brings to her patients is an incredible asset. In my practice I often encounter patients with severe foot and/or ankle problems. It is reassuring to have a colleague to refer patients in whom you have complete confidence.

Geraldine is able to get to the root of the problem with her extensive knowledge of the foot and how it works. She is also able to explain problems to her patients in a manner they easily understand. Her insightfulness into the foot and how it relates to the interaction of our bodies and environment is second to none. The publication of this much-needed book will help people understand the problems brought about by wearing incorrect footwear and its impact on the body. I will gladly recommend this book to patients. I have found it to be of great benefit to my patients to have a working relationship with Geraldine, and look forward to many more years of collaboration."

Keith H. Schaller, DC • Waterbury, VT
Internationally Certified Chiropractic Sports Physician

"Geraldine Villeneuve has written an educational and entertaining book touching on the history of shoes and delving into the theory of reflexology. The book comes alive with narratives of her personal experience using Structural Reflexology to treat clients.

I started seeing Geraldine about five years ago, after x-rays had ruled out a broken foot. She has kept my feet happy and healthy, allowing me to lead a very active life of hiking, dog agility, and dancing into my seventies."

L. von Trapp • Stowe, VT

"Geraldine employs a rare combination of science, skill and intuition in her work. She has created a therapeutic technique that has provided me more enduring relief from foot pain then several years of traditional and costly orthopedic intervention. Her structural reflexology work should be recognized as basic training for any practitioner of the healing arts and mandatory for orthopedic professionals!"

Suzanne Santarchangelo • Waterbury, VT
(55 year old bone cancer survivor with compromised calf and ankle functioning)

"I am a marathon runner. I first met Geraldine after an accident which resulted in a broken leg, broken ankle, multiple metatarsal fractures, and a greatly reduced range of motion. I saw immediate improvement after my first session with Geraldine. From that day forward, working with Geraldine became a very important part of my marathon training. I can't imagine running a marathon without her help."

Phyllis Arsenault-Berry • Waterbury, VT

"I was told by two podiatrists that I needed immediate surgery. One session with Geraldine and I could walk without pain. She has a unique understanding of the foot, and my feet are addicted! Don't know what I'd do without her…"

Jan Thouron • Middlesex, VT

Put Your Best Feet Forward

Exploring the causes and cures
of foot pain with Structural Reflexology®

By Geraldine Villeneuve

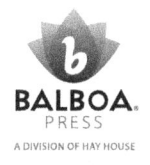

BALBOA
PRESS
A DIVISION OF HAY HOUSE

Copyright © 2017 Geraldine Villeneuve.

All rights reserved. No part of this book may be used or reproduced by any means, graphic, electronic, or mechanical, including photocopying, recording, taping or by any information storage retrieval system without the written permission of the author except in the case of brief quotations embodied in critical articles and reviews.

Put Your Best Feet Forward is written for the sole purpose of education and reference in personal practice. It is not to be used as a manual for instructional teaching by anyone other than the author. Any unauthorized copying will be considered an infringement of the copyright.

Balboa Press books may be ordered through booksellers or by contacting:

Balboa Press
A Division of Hay House
1663 Liberty Drive
Bloomington, IN 47403
www.balboapress.com
1 (877) 407-4847

Because of the dynamic nature of the Internet, any web addresses or links contained in this book may have changed since publication and may no longer be valid. The views expressed in this work are solely those of the author and do not necessarily reflect the views of the publisher, and the publisher hereby disclaims any responsibility for them.

The author of this book does not dispense medical advice or prescribe the use of any technique as a form of treatment for physical, emotional, or medical problems without the advice of a physician, either directly or indirectly. The intent of the author is only to offer information of a general nature to help you in your quest for emotional and spiritual well-being. In the event you use any of the information in this book for yourself, which is your constitutional right, the author and the publisher assume no responsibility for your actions.

Any people depicted in stock imagery provided by Thinkstock are models, and such images are being used for illustrative purposes only.
Certain stock imagery © Thinkstock.

Print information available on the last page.

ISBN: 978-1-5043-7323-4 (sc)
ISBN: 978-1-5043-7325-8 (hc)
ISBN: 978-1-5043-7324-1 (e)

Library of Congress Control Number: 2017900937

Balboa Press rev. date: 01/25/2017

Outside front cover design and greyscale version of the same in chapter 2 illustrated by Lisa Syverson.

Interior book illustrations: 6, 10, 12, and 18, were created in collaboration by Lisa Syverson and Geraldine Villeneuve.

All other interior illustrations by Geraldine Villeneuve unless stated otherwise.

Photos 1, 13, 14, 15, 16 by Geraldine Villeneuve
Photos 2, 3, 4, 5, 6, 7 by Dr. Phil Hoffman
Photos 10, 11, 12 by Thinkstock Getty Images

Author Photo by Kathleen Porter of North Productions, LLC, Westford, Vermont.

All rights reserved. Including the right of reproduction in whole or in part in any form.

STRUCTURAL REFLEXOLOGY® is a registered trademark of Geraldine Villeneuve.

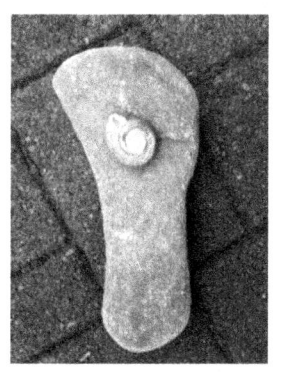

Photo 1
(See postscript for the story behind these fossils.)

Contents

Note ix
Acknowledgments xi
Preface xiii
Introduction xix

Chapter 1   Serendipity:
                How Reflexology Found Me 1
Chapter 2   Shoes 9
Chapter 3   The Foot Reflexology Map 17
Chapter 4   Reginald's Brain Reflexes 21
Chapter 5   The Relationship between the Arch of the Foot
                and the Spine 25
Chapter 6   The Gravitational Line 29
Chapter 7   What It Means to "Reflex" the Feet 33
Chapter 8   Theories about Foot Reflexology 37
Chapter 9   The Controversial Reflexology Map 41
Chapter 10 The Disappearing Little Toe 47
Chapter 11 Learning How to Walk Again 51
Chapter 12 Madeline 57
Chapter 13 Columns of the Foot 61
Chapter 14 The Cinderella Stepsister Complex:
                Understanding the Silent Breakdown of the Foot 67

Chapter 15 Flat Foot or "Fallen Arch?" 73
Chapter 16 The Nature of the Foot 81
Chapter 17 Long Foot Muscles and Their Reflex Sites 89
Chapter 18 The Calf Muscles and the Heart 107
Chapter 19 Arch Supports: "'To Be? or Not to Be?' That is
 the Question" 113
Chapter 20 Common Foot Problems Revealed 119

Conclusion 131
Postscript: The Fossils Story 135
Appendices 137
Works Cited 151
Index 153

Note

Put Your Best Feet Forward is about prevention and correction. It is not in any way intended to replace conventional medical therapy but to work as an adjunct and in partnership with the field of medicine to contribute to the greater good, health, and well-being of all people.

The Mission of *Put Your Best Feet Forward*:

- To revolutionize public awareness of the vital importance of healthy foot function

- To prioritize the feet to the A-list of anatomical importance

- To help others understand the feet are strong and capable and can take us through a lifetime of painless journeys without props

Acknowledgments

I want to thank my late mentor, teacher, and friend, Mr. William Rundquist, for introducing me to joint mobilization at the National Reflexology Conference in St. Louis, Missouri, and for taking me under his wing during the years I apprenticed with him.

My deepest gratitude and respect also goes to the pioneering works of Dr. John Martin Hiss, OD, and Dr. Simon Wikler, MD, for investing their lives to provide brilliant and masterful revelations and methods of restoring foot health without surgery, and for their unyielding commitment to their practice and teaching.

Their contributions to the field of foot function and correction of foot problems without surgery are enormously valuable. It is my honorable intention to respectfully expound on their work by providing clarity regarding how the feet impact the health of the rest of the body. Any misinterpretations in this book of Dr. Hiss and Dr. Wikler are entirely my own.

I also want to thank my students and clients who gave me the opportunity to master my profession as a Structural Reflexologist® by their interest in my skills and for their intelligent questions that always led me on a quest to learn more and give more.

My unending appreciation also goes to my editor, Julia Cicchetti, who demonstrated her tireless commitment to and passion for the successful production of *Put Your Best Feet Forward* by being there when I needed her expertise.

Lisa Syverson, my illustrator, felt like a friend from the moment we spoke. I am in awe of how easily our minds met in collaborating together. Her softness, beauty, and intelligence permeate the creative illustrations in *Put Your Best Feet Forward*, which speaks directly from who she is as a person.

I am grateful to internationally certified chiropractic sports physician Dr. Keith Schaller, DC, for his referrals and for recognizing structural reflexology as a valuable and professional healthcare modality.

I am thankful to my family and to my lovely mother, Virginia, whose incredible faith, strength, and leadership qualities have laid a foundation for me to cultivate the same in myself.

I very much appreciate the eternal loving support and patience of my husband, Neil, who was responsible for much of the technical aspect of producing *Put Your Best Feet Forward* and helped me to stretch beyond the edges of what I think I can do.

I dedicate this book to you in truth and in love.

Preface

Put Your Best Feet Forward will truly unlock the mystery of how reflexology works. After reading this book, you will find yourself saying, "Why didn't anyone tell me this before? It makes perfect sense!" You will feel compelled to release your beliefs regarding your feet and shoes, and you will elatedly turn the key that opens your own creative and personal treasure chest to becoming more comfortable in your own body.

Put Your Best Feet Forward will also release you from the pain and imprisonment caused by the foot-bound shoe, allowing you to relinquish your beliefs about shoe styles and foster a new mentality that supports the health and vitality of the foot in being strong and free, so you can be too.

I am so excited to take you on this gentle, powerful, and fantastic journey. Hang on; it's going to be a fun and inspiring ride!

What is reflexology?

Illustration 1

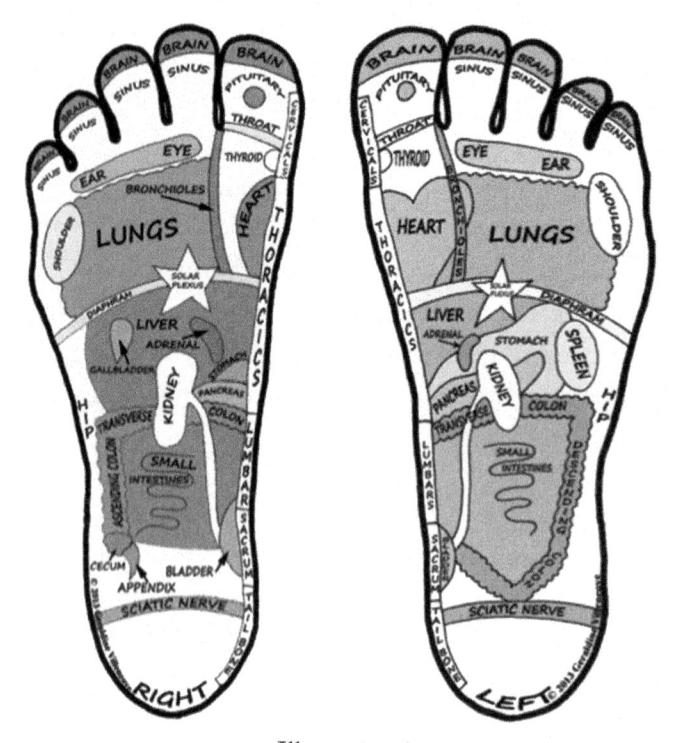

Illustration 1 portrays the bottom of the right and left foot with the organ system reflexes of the body.

Reflexology is a scientific practice and therapeutic art using microcosms (meaning the same, but miniature) of the body as an avenue to promote stress relief.

The main microcosms are specific to the feet, hands, and ears, whereby everything that is located on the left side of the body can be stimulated by a reflex area on the left foot, hand, or ear, and everything on the right side of the body can be stimulated by a reflex area on the right foot, hand, or ear.

Applied thumb and finger-walking techniques to areas called reflexes within these microcosms create a response in a corresponding part of the body.

Reflexology helps to soothe the nervous system, which in turn allows the body to relax and open up the circulatory processes. With improved circulation, oxygen and nutrition are delivered more efficiently while releasing stagnant waste products. As a result, the body feels refreshed, vital, and productive.

In her book *Art, Science & History*, Christine Issel describes that the origins of reflexology can be dated back to Ancient Egypt. A hieroglyph was found dated 2330 BC on the tomb of an Egyptian physician with inscriptions of the skills for which he was known, and one of these images is believed to be the first recording of reflexology.

Because of language barriers, during this time civilizations communicated through pictures and statues, which enabled countries such as India and Europe to learn this ancient healing art. Reflexology then reached North America in the late 1800s and was modernized in the early 1900s, when organ systems were more clearly mapped on the feet.

What Is Structural Reflexology®?

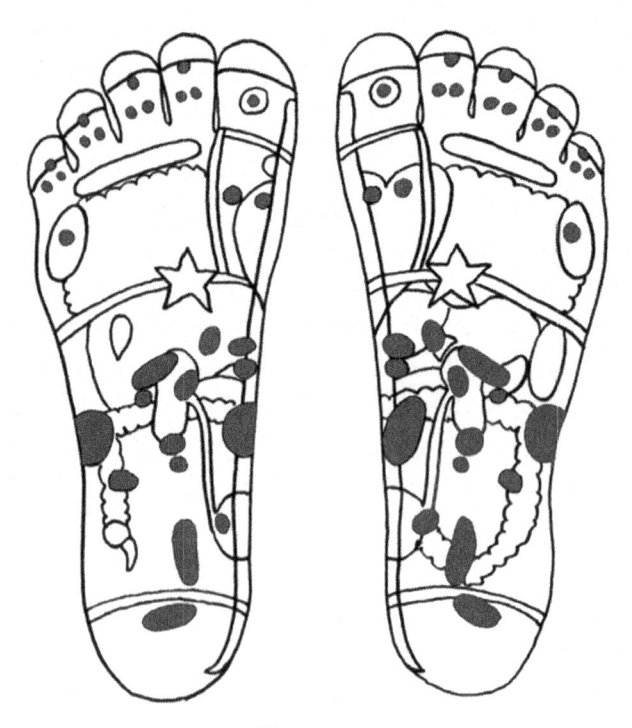

Illustration 2

The darkened areas in illustration 2 are sites of lower leg foot muscles as they attach to the bottom of the feet, with the reflexes associated with the body beneath.

Structural Reflexology® is the practice of integrating foot reflexology with anatomy, physiology, and kinesiology by using local and reflexive methods to release stress and compensation in the entire body.

Structural Reflexologists address tension sites on the feet as the product of local muscle and ligament strain while maintaining an understanding of how these sites of tension on the feet will impact the rest of the body.

Most individuals who seek the service of a Structural Reflexologist® are looking to relieve the stress of foot pain while benefiting from the calming effect of reflexology. The nervous system speaks loudly when it comes to foot discomfort because of the thousands of nerve endings in the feet that make them extra sensitive. Usually the person seeking out reflexology has tried everything, and Structural Reflexology® becomes their last resort, and it leaves them wondering in the end why they didn't go this route to begin with.

The Aim of Structural Reflexology®

- Assess the feet to discover the cause of the disorder.
- Identify tension sites in the foot and leg that create inappropriate weight distribution and compensation in the upper parts of the body.
- Improve foot alignment and function to decrease inflammation throughout the foot and body.
- Bring the foot back to a stage that is comfortable.

Introduction

My Memories of Feet

Feet have fascinated me ever since I can remember touching my own.

One of my earliest recollections of feet was while I was an infant. I can vividly recall feeling pure joy at the sight of my feet and toes. I remember thinking, *How funny looking are those! What are those things that stick out and wiggle?* I remember laughing at the wonder of it.

The glimmer of shiny patent leather shoes at Easter is a memorable anchor as well. They were not very comfortable, but they were pretty, and I wore them with pride in all their discomfort. I used to fantasize about taking the blades off my white leather skates and wearing them as shoes. There was something about that sound on the floor that exhilarated me.

Likewise, wearing my mother's, and my friends' mothers', high heels was a real treat as we played dress up. My ankles would bend sideways in my attempt to move in them, and my little feet were not strong enough to navigate my body in them. I figured out that scuffing along the floor helped to keep them on, but I soon became bored and abandoned them. In a way I suppose, like passing the baton, this could have been the initiation to the follies of the long, pointed shoe style for my generation. My need to run, jump, and play led me to prefer being barefoot to wearing any kind of shoes, and this freedom of movement became very physically ingrained in me.

Most of my childhood years were spent running around barefoot on asphalt and grassy areas, and my feet were often grass-stained and dirty. I felt free this way. I loved the feel of the grass and my feet against the surface of the earth as my uncle Ernest (who used to call me "grasshopper") encouraged me to dance, twirl, and tumble on the dewy grass while my folks watched *The Lawrence Welk Show*.

By the time I was eight, I became a gymnast and learned the value of the unencumbered foot when it comes to balance and precision, especially on the balance beam. Now I understand why my shoulders became strong from using all of my toes for balance.

After my father's long days at work, I felt inclined to rub his feet, which he gladly accepted. I thought it would help him relax and feel better after the stressors of his job. He was providing for my mother and twelve children, after all, and I felt this was how I could contribute. I noticed they were ticklish, red in spots, and hot. He would pull them back and wince at times because of the sensitivity, but he seemed to like it all the same.

I also recall how oddly stiff they were, and not until I learned about the relationship of foot function and shoes did I realize that my father must have been wearing the wrong size shoe for years!

Had I known then what I know now about shoes and foot motion, I would have seen the signs of rigidity and points of redness on his feet as symptoms of foot strain that resulted from wearing shoes that did not fit correctly. I would have been able to help him regain the power and vitality of his feet so he could release the tension that was building in his body. By simply changing his shoe size, he would have had a chance to wear shoes that allowed the arches of his feet to move, and with this easy change, his chronic back pain would have been eliminated. But we didn't know the impact shoes have on the body and how easily the feet tolerate being bound.

He died at the early age of sixty-one of heart failure, and yes, I often wonder if my father died from complications of restricted blood-flow caused by wearing the wrong size shoe. It made sense when people said at my father's funeral they remember seeing him always running to get from here to there. I remembered this, too. I strongly believe it was because he could not walk due to the intensity of the muscle and ligament tension built up in his shoe-bound feet.

It saddens me to think about it, and I suppose this event has made me more determined to educate the public about the importance of vital and healthy feet.

Chapter 1

Serendipity: How Reflexology Found Me

It was the summer of 1981. I had just finished my sophomore year of college and was much in need of a job. Given my studies in therapeutic health and physical education, I decided to take a job as a nurse's aide in a nursing home. At the age of nineteen, I willingly entered into the world of geriatrics and was happy to have a job.

Some of my responsibilities entailed keeping the residents comfortable and feeding and bathing those who needed assistance. I was also given the job of taking blood pressure and pulses, recording the intake of fluids and output of urine, and testing sugar levels for those suffering with diabetes.

As the summer continued, my knowledge and responsibilities grew. I got to know my patients and greatly enjoyed the warm and simple exchanges that occurred as these relationships developed.

In the process of carrying out my responsibilities, I couldn't shake the phenomenon of the appearance of most of my patients' feet. I referred to them as "mushroom-capped" feet because this is what they looked like when it came time for me to take their shoes off. The tops of their feet looked swollen and bulbous, while their toes and heels were shriveled and slight. It bothered me deeply, and I instinctively washed and rubbed their feet and watched their faces melt with relief as their feet relaxed into a more normal shape. I felt happy to be able to provide comfort in this way.

One midsummer day I was perusing a book that described many ways to heal the body, and I came upon a diagram that illustrated the organs of the body drawn on the bottoms of the feet. Both amused and amazed at the absurdity of this image, my interest was piqued, and I could not let this pass by. I had to prove or disprove this and was intent on figuring it out.

I copied the page, brought the diagram with me to work, and began investigating the possibility of its truth.

Illustration 3

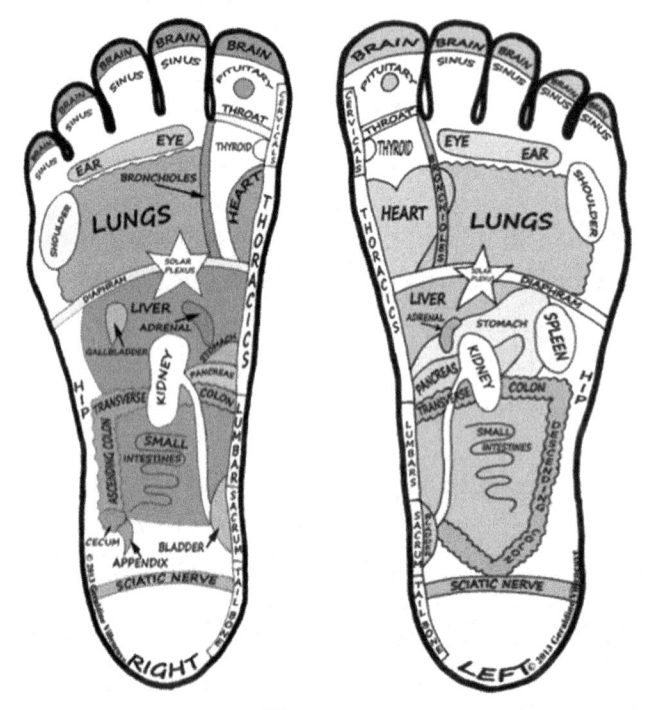

Illustration 3: This foot reflexology map is one that I personally produced from tracing my own feet. The diagram I saw in the early 1980s was not so detailed.

Having access to the medical charts, and with permission from my patients, I was able to associate the image of the foot map to *their* feet. With my thumbs, I palpated sites on their feet to investigate correlations with their medical chart. For example, if a patient was experiencing constipation, I palpated the areas where the map cited as the reflex area to the colon. I would then compare this texture with that of another patient's foot who was not experiencing constipation. I was amazed how tactilely different they were.

The possibilities of learning about this intrigued me to no end, and my patients loved it. With permission from the charge nurse, I began to take a few of my patients' pulses and blood pressures before and after I palpated sites on their feet and noted a significant and positive change in the measurement. I even took the opportunity to test blood-sugar levels to see if reflexology could influence pancreatic function by decreasing the sugar levels in urine, and I was thrilled to see that it did.

I began to see obvious changes in the dispositions of the patients I was working with over that summer. I knew reflexology was benefiting them, but it was still very mysterious to me, and like a new best friend, I took this newfound knowledge with me wherever I went to test it and to learn from it. I bought every reflexology book I could get my hands on, and in my spare time throughout the remainder of college, I practiced on my friends and family and read all I could about reflexology.

As part of completing my bachelor of science degree, I was required to fulfill an internship, which I chose to do in the orthopedic division at the Children's Hospital in Boston. My job was to provide therapy to the patients through play and activity. I loved this job and am so thankful for the experience of working in this superb establishment.

While I was there, reflexology again beckoned to me, this time to the autism division as I passed this floor on my way to the orthopedic unit.

I couldn't help but think how wonderful it would be if reflexology could create a calming effect for children with autism who were confined to cribs, waiting to have dental work. With permission from my supervisor and the charge nurse on duty, I was able to calm a wonderful child with autism with a ten-minute reflexology session. The two of us then peacefully took a walk in the garden courtyard below without incident. This event was a topic for conversation for quite a while after, as typically this child was not able to focus long enough to stand still. Needless to say, I was thrilled.

Toward the end of my internship, my supervisor asked me what I planned on presenting during the required public education forum at the hospital. I froze. At the time I was not comfortable speaking in public, and my head became foggy in my attempt to figure out what I could talk about for forty-five minutes.

After a few days of thinking it through, I bravely asked my supervisor if she would allow me to talk about reflexology. Since she was privy to my extracurricular reflexology sessions with children with autism at the hospital, she acquiesced to this idea with excitement about learning more. I then asked if I could demonstrate on her, and amused and delighted, she agreed.

The day of the presentation soon came, and so did a "eureka moment." While speaking and demonstrating the reflexology technique I had developed over the last two and a half years, I found myself repeatedly palpating a particular raised texture on my supervisor's hand that was a reflex site associated with the ear, until she shrieked, "*Ouch!*"

My face reddened, and I apologized for hurting her, but she promptly stopped me midsentence and said, "No you don't understand—my ear has been plugged up for two years, and it just popped open!" She thanked me, and the audience "oohed" and "ahhed," and they were almost as amazed as I. It worked, and I didn't even know there was a problem! Needless to say, I received an A+ on this presentation.

After receiving my bachelor's of science degree in therapeutic studies, I took a job in Vermont as an activities therapist in the Psychiatric Division of the Brattleboro Retreat. I was a therapist on a treatment team for both schizophrenia and eating disorders. Here I led and co-led various activities for the patients' therapeutic involvement.

After careful planning, and with the collective approval of the treatment teams, I introduced and led a therapeutic activity called, "Learn How to Do Reflexology" for patient participation. The effect of the class on the patients was much greater than I anticipated, so it was agreed to keep "Learn How to Do Reflexology" on the schedule as a regular activity option.

This once-a-week class became very popular, and it was always at capacity. Because of this there were two nurses or other staff present in the room as well.

The patients learned an abbreviated version of reflexology, its benefits, and how to give and receive a session. It was remarkable to see the transformation on the faces of these folks as they filed out of the room looking dignified and serene.

One of the psychiatrists heartily remarked to me at rounds, "What are you doing in there? The patients come out of the room and act as if they have been given a calming drug."

I noticed many of the doctors and nurses observing through the window during these classes, and each week the staff began to compete for the chance to be in the room to participate.

Little did I know reflexology was becoming my obsession. I was becoming an authority on the subject because of all the questions people asked, and if I didn't have the answer, I'd research it. Invitations began to pour in to speak in various forums about reflexology and to be the staff reflexologist during health symposiums.

In 1986 I participated in a life-changing course in New York City on the subject of how to improve your relationship with yourself in order to improve your relationships with others. After completing this four-day seminar, I felt pleasantly raw and fatigued with enlightenment as I, and the throngs of other people who indulged in this fabulous workshop, trailed out of the auditorium. Suddenly, however, someone accidently knocked into the back of my knees, causing me to tumble to the floor and drop all of my notes and belongings. One of the participants assisted me upright and helped me gather my things as we introduced ourselves and spoke of where we lived and worked.

During our brief encounter, something in me spontaneously interjected, "Have you ever heard of reflexology?" Her eyes widened as she replied, "Heard of it! I have a school of reflexology right here in Manhattan!" I told her I never knew there was such a thing as a school for reflexology. I of course enrolled in and received a master's of reflexology certification and stayed on afterward to complete a teacher's apprenticeship program.

I officially received my master's of reflexology certificate in 1989. Until that point reflexology was a side interest, and I never entertained the idea of making a living at it. I then opened a private reflexology practice in Brattleboro, Vermont, and I began to incorporate what I had been teaching myself since 1981 with what I learned in New York. My practice soon bloomed as the reflexology results spoke for themselves.

The following year I decided to move to Seattle, and I was unnerved to hear that in order to practice reflexology in the state of Washington, I needed to have a massage therapy license. The penalty would be a criminal record if I dared practice without this license. After talking with the health department in Olympia, I decided it was moot to think I could change this law, even after passionately clarifying that reflexology and massage therapy are two entirely different entities, and that in my experience and conversations with many massage therapists, most knew very little about reflexology, so why was it under the massage therapy umbrella? I was sent out the door with, "Sorry, but that's the law."

Back to school I went, and I received my massage practitioner's license at the Brenneke School of Massage with a specialization in treatment for injuries. I was proud of my accomplishment, for the massage curriculum proved to be an academic challenge, and I learned a lot more about the human body and how to help people recover from trauma.

After graduating from massage school, I immediately opened my reflexology practice and decided to teach. I named my business Seattle Reflexology and Massage Center. The name rolled off my tongue, and I had come to realize my reflexology practice became a life unto itself. I was the conduit for its manifestation and growth, and I was honored to be the facilitator.

I was hired to be on staff at the Brenneke School of Massage as the faculty reflexology instructor. The introductory course to reflexology was a hit, and so was my advanced reflexology course. "I want to learn more," was a popular response, and before long I produced a well-attended and successful master's of reflexology certification series.

This certification series was born out of a culmination of experiences from my personal adventures in learning and practicing reflexology; my formal reflexology training; and my local, national, and international reflexology involvement. The reflexology conferences I attended fed my unending desire to learn more, teach more, and assimilate it all to bring back to my students. In fact, when I was particularly fascinated with the subject, I would invite the speaker to teach his or her method at my school. These speaker invitations became the standard for the school curriculum, which increased the school's education hours and began to form the center's larger purpose: an international hub for reflexology training.

In the interim between my teaching and practice, I was one of a small panel of reflexologists who met with the purpose of learning what other schools of reflexology were teaching around the country to come up with a set of national educational standards for school accreditation. We named this organization the "American Commission of Accreditation for Reflexology Education and Training," or ACARET for short.

I also hadn't dropped the ball on the health department in Washington regarding the status of reflexology training being governed by the Massage Therapy Department, and with the encouragement of some reflexology friends and colleagues, namely Christine Issel and Bill Flocco, we started a committee to change the law. It involved getting through many legal snarls and constant vigilance on everyone's part.

My participation was in the birth and developmental stages of creating a state reflexology association for Washington. The baton was then passed to my apprentice, Lisa Hensell, who purchased the Seattle Reflexology and Massage Center in 1999. Her passion for reflexology spoke through her perseverance, leadership, and administration skills as she and our fellow reflexology colleagues continued to pave the way for reflexology to become what it is now: a professional and independent entity in the state of Washington! Hooray!

Reflexology still remains fresh and lively in my life in Vermont. I continue to engage in reflexology practice, teaching, and learning, and I realize now more than ever the very organic meaning of the word and the truth of how it works. This is what this book is about.

Chapter 2

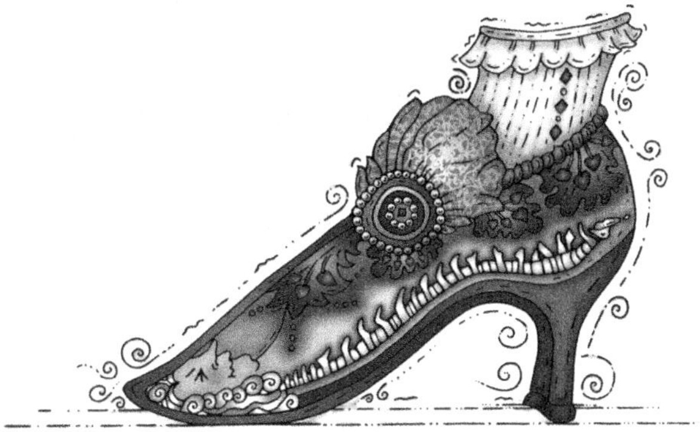

Illustration 4

Shoes

The popular phrase "put your best foot forward" has been circulating throughout literature since as early as 1495.

Written a century later, Shakespeare used a form of that expression in *King John* saying, "Nay, but make haste; the better foot before."

During this period, the shoe of desire, worn mostly by royalty, was very narrow, with a pointed toe. The vast majority of people were peasants who spent their entire lives barefoot, as shoes were expensive and only hand made. Though the translation of this phrase was meant to imply "do your best," in my opinion this phrase has literal meaning in that the majority of the world's population has foot problems. What on earth is the cause of this? Most of the time I seem to find the answer in shoes.

To this day, the style and yes, cost of one's shoes communicates so much about the wearer: personality, affluence, prestige, and sex appeal.

There is no arguing the importance shoes play in our lives. The style of shoes, however, has become more valued than function and often errs on the side of costumey rather than protective and functional.

For most of society the brain has been stuck in a seductive, stylish shoe passed on from the days of King Louis XIV, who wore the pointed-toe, heeled shoe that differentiated the peasants from those of affluence. It was considered a political privilege to wear these types of shoes, and those who had access to the king's court were more likely able to afford them.

Eventually King Louis passed an edict that only those who were already admitted to court were allowed to wear them. The heels of these shoes were often painted red to signify that royalty and nobility didn't dirty their heels, and the heel itself signified that they were ready to "crush the enemies of the state at their feet" (Forbes, 2016).

I sometimes wonder about the look of King Louis's feet and why he was so intent on wearing this tapered-style shoe. Why hold the toes hostage by bridling them tightly together? Was it an effort to hide them, cover them up, and disguise his pain with a bow-topped shoe?

Sadly, I happen to think this attitude is still held by many people who have deformed their feet by their shoe choices.

Shoes were originally measured in barleycorns for length, and they were made from the same tools used in Egypt since the fourteenth century until the modern manufactured shoe was developed in the mid-1800s following the invention of the sewing machine. This enabled material to be fastened to the platform of the shoe more efficiently.

The production of the modern manufactured shoe offered the public a way to afford shoes at a reasonable price. It was all the rage!

However, the essential difference between hand-sewn shoes and modern, manufactured shoes was that the right and left shoes were equally matched in the manufactured shoe. With hand-sewn shoes, the cobbler took many measurements into consideration in sizing each shoe individually to match the shape and contour of each foot. Most people have two different-size feet, and therefore, the majority of people who wear the modern shoe are forcing their feet to conform to shoes that do not fit.

In a more practical light, the heeled boot or shoe once served the purpose of keeping one's foot from sliding forward in the stirrup as soldiers galloped on their horses during the Civil War, and today they are still a necessity for horseback-riding ranchers and cattle handlers.

However, like the flip-flop, the heeled and pointed-toe cowboy boot has diverged from its original intent and is worn as a statement of everyday fashion. This boot was not meant to pound the pavement or to dance in, which would be strenuous to the feet as the shape of this shoe folds the foot and toes, making it awkward to bear weight.

I used to think the bowlegged appearance of many horseback riders was because their legs took the shape of the barreled back of their horse, until I saw what they commonly wear on their feet: pointed cowboy boots. The people wearing the pointed-toe-box boot essentially stuff and manipulate the delicate, yet forgiving, tissue of the feet into these boots that are shaped nothing like feet.

Above the imprisoned feet, the knees and hips distort as they struggle to adjust to the binding and bowing of the feet below. Subsequently, the ligaments that keep the knees and hips aligned become irritated and arthritic, preventing the normal, correct hinging of the knee and fluid hip movement. The ligaments of the foot designed to balance the body in space weaken and lose their elasticity and ability to keep the bones of the foot in place.

The immobilizing effect of this boot significantly prevents the long foot muscles from doing their job of moving the foot, and they settle into a state of lethargy, while the ligaments of the foot that ordinarily help balance the body now woefully underperform their function from their leather bindings. Consequently, the entire body is left to seek alternative routes to stabilize and move. This draws energy from the larger, upper body muscle groups to assist and thus reduces the body's potential to compensatory and debilitating dysfunction in its struggle to initiate graceful and flowing movement.

Recently, one of my clients with foot pain exclaimed with pride that her feet had actually gotten smaller over the years. Incidentally, she wore pointed-toe cowboy boots on a daily basis. After measuring her feet, her affect presented a bewildered disappointment when I revealed she was wearing shoes two sizes too small.

"But these boots are so comfortable!" she said with deflated enthusiasm. I explained that it was just an illusion that her feet were smaller. I further explained that, in fact, the muscles of her feet became atrophied from inactivity while adapting to this style and fashion of boot.

The initial warning signs of pain and discomfort from wearing these boots became overshadowed by the desire to wear them. Meanwhile, the muscles and joints of the feet are so resilient it could take five to ten years before they can no longer adapt to being bound. Even though the foot stops complaining, the tension caused from wearing shoes that do not fit the shape of the feet creates curious compensations throughout the body, disguising the progression of foot deformity. Once a joint in the foot locks under this accumulated pressure, the warning signal becomes real, and one is left with a foot problem. This is what happened to my client.

The boots had weakened and deformed her feet—yes, in the way foot-binding is designed to do—and the muscles of her feet had atrophied from underuse and abuse, giving them the appearance of being much smaller. She returned a couple months later wearing new shoes, two sizes larger and with a wide toe box. She had a youthful sparkle in her eye, tilted her foot with pride, and said, "I love them— and they are so comfortable!" Her foot pain had subsided completely.

After carefully measuring over 150,000 feet with his classifootometer, Dr. John Martin Hiss, OD, discovered there are three types of feet:

1. 70 percent of this group measured longer arches than their toe-to-heel measurement (short toes).
2. 20 percent had the same measurement in the arch as they did toe-to-heel.
3. 10 percent of this group measured a shorter arch and a longer toe-to-heel (long toes). (1949)
   (See Appendix C for "How to Measure the Feet.")

Based on Dr. Hiss's findings, 80 percent of his patients were wearing the wrong size shoe (1949). Shoes are not designed to accommodate the arch-size discrepancies, which explains why we are a culture experiencing a multitude of foot problems.

In his effort to remedy the issue of shoes causing foot problems, the late Dr. Simon Wikler, doctor of surgical podiatry, designed the Wikler Shoe by Buster Brown. He strongly believed the design of the manufactured shoe was responsible for the majority of foot problems and considered this issue a chronic, widespread "dis-ease" bigger than most degenerative diseases combined. His passion for this work became most intense when he attributed his mother's early death to the degenerative irritation from the stress put upon her entire body from her shoes.

In his studies of foot function and shoes, Dr. Wikler noted that since the modern manufactured shoe industry was born, it also increased the need for chiropractors and psychiatrists, no doubt because of the strain and increased pressure shoes impress upon the bones and our precious nerves and blood supply, not to mention the excessive exertion it takes to move a foot in a shoe that does not fit (1953).

He determined that a properly fitted shoe is essential for healthy biomechanics of the foot. He emphasized that flexible shoes promote strength and vitality and encourage natural foot movement. He discouraged wearing rigid shoes that inhibit the essential movement of the arch.

Dr. Wikler also necessitated that at least three measurements be considered for proper shoe fitting using a Brannock Measuring Device (which is still considered to be the most accurate), and that if a shoe was off even one-sixteenth of an inch it would cause enough strain to throw off the delicate balance of the foot (1953).

I first learned of Dr. Wikler and Dr. Hiss from reflexologist Mr. William (Bill) Rundquist at a national reflexology conference. Bill was one of the guest speakers and gave a very provocative speech on foot function. He relayed valuable foot-assessment information he gathered from the archives of Dr. Wikler, as well as that on foot-joint mobilization he received from the founder of this method, podiatrist and reflexologist Dr. Harvey Lampell, who was a student of Dr. Hiss. The message was clear: shoes matter and are very influential factors in the health and wellbeing of the entire body, and the feet are the gateway to managing the health of the body, mind, and spirit.

As I listened to Bill speak, the doors of my mind released a flood of connections regarding the feet as a microcosm of the body. Foot reflexology and foot function were converging seamlessly in my mind as a natural partnership in their connectedness.

In my excitement I could hardly contain myself. Everything I struggled with in making sense of how foot reflexology works suddenly became clear. This information was the missing link, and I suddenly recognized foot reflexology coming full circle from its Egyptian genesis. It all made sense, and my head whirled with the magnificence of it all.

I breathed with elation when Bill agreed to be a regular faculty member at my reflexology school in Seattle, where I began to apprentice with him over the next three years.

My years of experience, understanding, and practice laid the groundwork for teaching reflexology combined with foot assessment and kinesiology into a model that fit into my scope of practice, which I called passive foot mobilization. While honing in on this specific approach of releasing muscle, joint, and ligament tension, I was beginning to understand its more direct relationship with reflexology on the whole. The more rigid the foot, the more rigid the body becomes; the more flexible the foot, the more flexible the body becomes. This answered my lifelong question about feet being a microcosm of the body, a perfect match of the whole: "so with the feet, so with the body."

Bill Rundquist was exceptional in his practice as a foot-joint mobilization specialist, and people flew in from all over the country to see him because of his success in alleviating foot problems. His approach was very scientific and related mostly to foot function. I admired him greatly, and my desire to learn from him was boundless. In studying with Bill, I realized he did not consider the same correlation of how reflexology and foot joint mobilization worked together as I did.

For example, Bill was suffering with a shoulder cuff injury and proclaimed during one of the classes he was teaching that one would not be able to find the reflex to this injury on a microcosmic level on his foot. Surprised by his statement, I jovially challenged this assertion. He invited me to enlighten him, and voila, there I found it on the bottom of his foot near the little toe (the reflex area of the shoulder) and in surprise of this discovery, he said, "Ouch!"

I studied the relationship of reflexology and foot-joint mobility with every session I gave and became convinced that the two are inseparable, and that one was birthed from the other, and thus Structural Reflexology® was born.

Chapter 3
The Foot Reflexology Map

Illustration 5

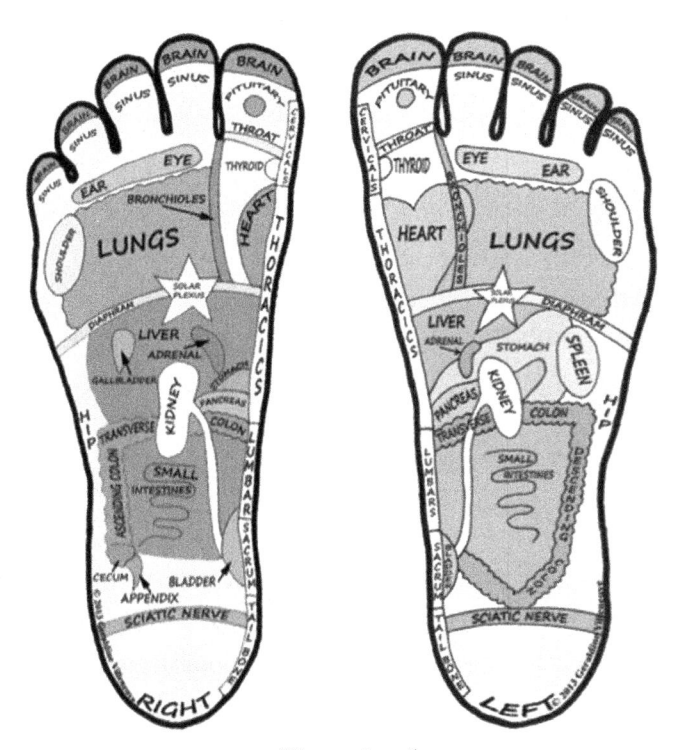

Illustration 5: The images above are the bottom of the right and left feet and the corresponding reflexes.

The foot reflexology map is more than the image of organs and glands drawn on the bottom of the feet. This popular, and easily misunderstood, map is an important blueprint of where imbalances can occur in the body based on the health of the feet, and is influenced by how well the feet articulate with movement.

Correct weight-bearing on the lateral side of the foot and the healthy spring-action of the medial arch of the foot will set the tone for organized movement up and out the spine, with the potential to invigorate and promote appropriate neural activity to the glands and organs of the body. If there is misalignment in the bones of the feet, the affected area will directly impose the need for compensation upon the structures above this weakness, thus impacting the organ systems that are stimulated by the initiation of movement in specific parts of the foot.

A professional reflexologist recognizes that together the feet represent a perfect match of an individual's entire body. He or she can truly see the feet as the body's microcosmic equal.

With specific thumb and finger-walking techniques performed on an individual's feet, the reflexologist's goal is to relieve stress by calming the nervous system via the thousands of nerve endings found on the bottom of the feet, thus promoting relaxation, improved blood flow throughout the body, and the restoration of balance.

Those seeking relief from foot pain have reported wonderful success with Structural Reflexology®, while also sharing how other ailments in their body, such as ringing in the ears, chronic sinus blockages, and vertigo, for example, have completely resolved as well.

The goal of the Structural Reflexologist® is to detect *why* and *where* compensation sets into the body based on foot alignment and function, and correlates this with their knowledge of the feet as a microcosm of the body. The Structural Reflexologist® seeks to correct foot problems by seeking the *cause* of painful symptoms. First by assessing foot structure, alignment, and joint and muscle tension, and then with intent, purpose, and precision, utilizing reflexology, massage techniques, and gentle traction, to bring the feet back to a stage that is comfortable and functional, thus relieving symptoms presenting in other parts of the body caused by compensation.

The feet are forgiving and can adapt to the abnormal circumstances forced upon them for decades before pain sets in, if at all. In fact, a person can live an entire lifetime without foot pain even if there are dislocations in the feet, as long as the joints of the feet remain unlocked. The upper body may suffer, however, and present pain because of the compensation necessary to move the body with feet that have become functionally dysfunctional.

The force of strain that feet endure will change the balance of the mechanism of the feet and inhibit normal foot function. The great news is this is all avoidable and correctable given the right size and style shoe.

Chapter 4
Reginald's Brain Reflexes

Illustration 6

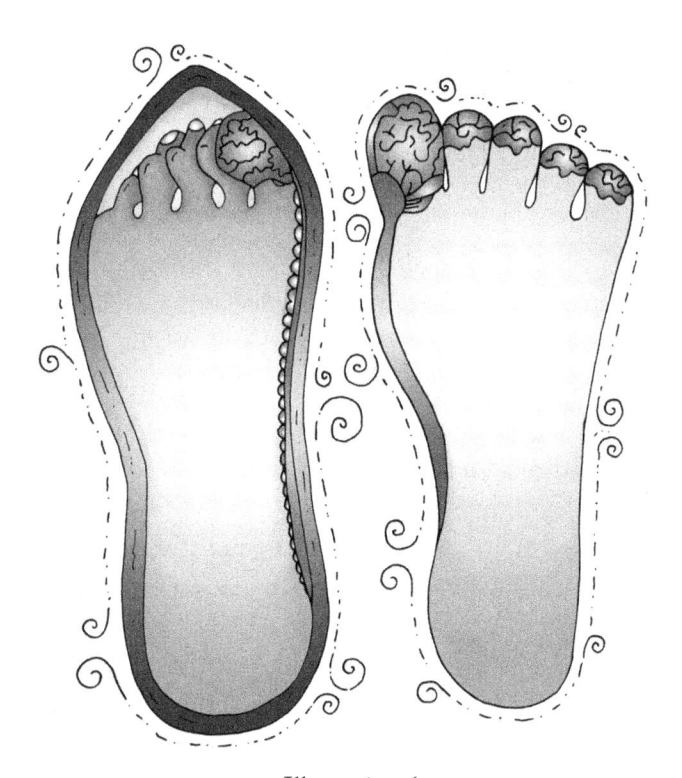

Illustration 6: Left image is a foot in a shoe that is too small putting pressure against the brain reflexes. Right image is a foot without pressure against the brain reflex sites.

According to Dr. Wikler, only 5 percent of foot deformities exhibit pain. As mentioned previously, Dr. Wikler spoke of the probability of developing degenerative issues by wearing incorrectly sized shoes (1953). This information pierced my heart when a client was referred to me for reflexology by his psychiatrist for stress-relief, and she disclosed to me that he had suicidal tendencies. As with all my sessions, I approached this one with an open mind and heart.

When Reginald (his name has been changed here for the purposes of confidentiality), by far one of my favorite people, entered my office, he divulged he had thought of jumping off a bridge on his way to his appointment with me, and that most of the time he stayed home because of these dreadful inclinations. I expressed my sincere appreciation that he came in to receive reflexology from me. He had no complaints of foot pain, but I noticed his toes were curled under, and the tips and middle joint of each of his toes were callused. I made a mental note that the toes represent reflex areas for the brain and head.

As with every new client, I then proceeded to measure his feet. He told me he wore a size 11 shoe, but after measuring each foot, we were both astounded to find his feet measured size 14! The possibility that his symptoms of suicidal ideation developed from wearing shoes that were too small startled me. His toes were crunched and curled into shoes that were three sizes too small.

With further assessment, Reginald's feet were stiff and showing very little articulation, almost as if each foot were one solid bone.

Working with Reginald that day was like releasing fireworks at the fair, and after this session, with an uplifted tone, he said he felt wonderful and was going on a shopping mission to purchase bigger shoes. (We decided that a 12 shoe size would be a good start.)

He received two reflexology sessions a week, and by the end of one month, Reginald stated he was feeling less suicidal and decided to venture out of his condo and take a dance class. We decided it was time to increase his shoe size to 13. His toes were uncurling daily as his joints began to articulate and find their function again. (A process that can be somewhat uncomfortable for a short time.)

As his toes unfurled, I witnessed Reginald emerging from the chains that bound his physical prosperity as he continued with his dance class and became more and more social. During one of his sessions, he surprised me by saying he decided to open up a latte stand at a popular film festival.

Eventually his reflexology appointments lessened to once every three weeks, then once a month, and by the end of four months, Reginald fit his now-straightened toes comfortably into his size 14 shoe and was as social as ever.

Reginald was involved in other modalities of therapy as well as reflexology, but I could clearly link the small shoes he wore as a contributor to this destructive behavior. In weight-bearing motion, the natural articulation of the toes allows the head and neck to move freely with the flow of movement of the cervical spine where the cranial nerves are housed. In my opinion Reginald's brain reflexes (his toes) were being under-stimulated because his toes were not able to move in his size 11 shoes.

This caused an extreme handicap in mobility when he walked or moved, leaving the heavy head and neck vulnerable, hence the need to compensate. In motion, without the strength of the toes to rely on, the head and neck will retreat back into the shoulders, similar to what a turtle does to get back into his shell. The muscular tension created by this compensation can very likely diminish nerve and blood supply to the head and brain and could account for his depression.

As far as local implications, the foot suffers greatly, and the thirty-eight foot joints that articulate and balance the body become challenged, though often do not exhibit pain, and this is why the feet are not usually taken into account as the cause of degenerative issues in the body.

Eighteen years later, I contacted Reginald. He spoke of some of the many accomplishments he has achieved, including training in reflexology, acupuncture, and zero balancing. Recently he has walked and bicycled the five hundred–mile Camino de Santiago and is now comfortably wearing size 15 boots!

Chapter 5

The Relationship between the Arch of the Foot and the Spine

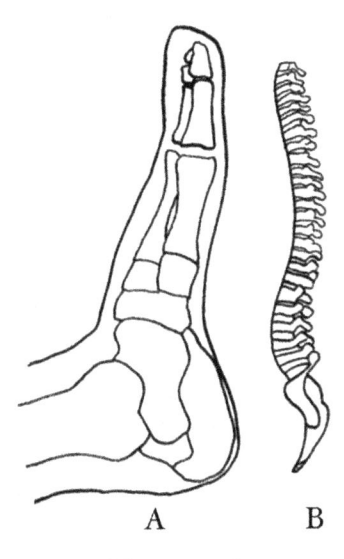

Illustration 7

The brilliant Dr. John Martin Hiss, MD, DO, was a very influential teacher in the development of my Structural Reflexology® practice. In his book *New Feet for Old* (1933), he eloquently describes how he learned the feet are designed very similarly to the mechanics of a clock, working in perfect tandem and precision. He remarked that the finely tuned and balanced clock would break and stop immediately from forceful pressures against its relationship of movement. This is not unlike the abused, bound foot. Unlike the clock, however, even if the mechanics of the foot break down, the brain will find another way to move the body. It will override normal foot function, and with the sheer willpower to get from here to there, draw on the energy of the larger muscles groups to move the body. Compensation then exhibits in posture changes, and neural and endocrine activity become confused.

In my thirty-five years of experience, I have observed and concluded that the degree of curves in the arch of the foot are an exact blueprint of the degree of curves in the spine of any given individual, and every incremental movement the arch of the foot makes creates a catalyst of movement for each segment of the vertebrae during locomotion. Because of this, one can isolate where tension in the back is brewing by assessing the tension in the arch of the foot, and vice versa, tension in certain areas of the spine can direct me to specific areas in the arch of the foot that have become tense.

The movement of the arch initiates a waving motion up the body and through the spinal column to the brain. This powerful energy produced by the unencumbered arch of the foot keeps the nervous system feeding efficient and appropriate signals to the muscles, glands, and organs, and fosters healthy blood and lymph flow throughout the body when walking.

When one chooses to impede the movement of the arch of the foot by wearing rigid, inflexible shoes, or worse, high heels, the arch of the foot becomes inert and will soon yield confusion in the muscles that move the feet and body because of their binding effect on the foot. These types of shoes cast the feet in an abnormal position, creating great strain on the foot and the rest of the body, and in particular, the spine.

I am convinced that those who wear high heels are demonstrating a self-imposed circus act. The energy and effort it takes to wear shoes like this, much less get around in them, is substantial. The power of movement is no longer coming from the feet but is drawn from other parts of the body, especially the hips and shoulders. This explains the dramatic swaying of the hips you often see in the high heel-wearer, or occasionally the opposite is true and they tiptoe or shuffle to keep balance. The exaggerated effort to move the body becomes more obvious when the feet can no longer perform under normal conditions, especially as we age.

The distorted movement created by wearing high heels will transmit the impact of one's weight from the heel of the foot to balls of foot. The design of the high heel inhibits the crucial function of the arch of the foot, which is to absorb the impact of body weight as the foot carries the body. The impact of 98 percent of body weight is imposed on the balls of the feet with every step; this therefore eliminates the arches' natural buffer. Instead of a wave-like, propelling motion, the high heel forces a *heel-to-toe* impact that encourages varying degrees of compression of the knees, hips, low back, and neck. Not only will the skeletal body break down, but the internal workings of the body also become irritated and misplaced by the postural deviations caused by trying to move the body against gravity while wearing this type of shoe. (See illustration 8 A and B.)

Illustration 8

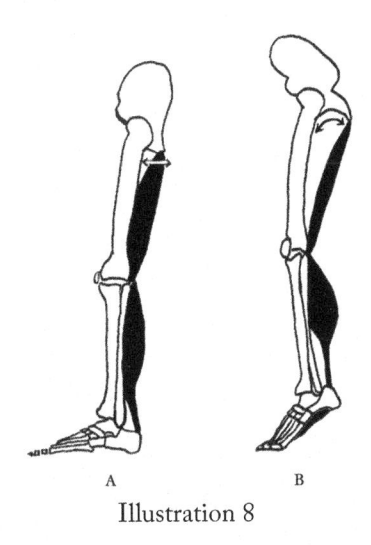

Illustration 8: Image A shows the outside of the leg and its relaxed muscle attachments from the heel to the knee, and from the knee to the pelvis. Image B demonstrates strain of these muscles while propped up in a high heel.

The fallout from wearing any shoes that do not allow the feet to perform their normal function may never be traced to shoes. The feet are so adaptable to all sorts of abuse that functional foot disorders may brew for years before ever being detected or linked to the wearer's past or present use of shoes. In other words, shoes may covertly cause functional foot disorders and allow the foot to move without causing pain to the feet. Chronic use of dysfunctional shoes, however, will create compensation throughout the rest of the body and communicate strain elsewhere. This may even cause degenerative issues difficult to trace back to the misaligned foot.

Structural foot disorders, on the other hand, speak to locked joints in the feet, which translates to locked joints throughout the body and actual foot pain. This condition is more overt and easier to assess because pain presents in the foot as slight to extreme foot-joint tension. Despite the pain, this can be a more fortunate scenario for those afflicted with foot problems as often the issue is addressed before compensation progresses into more serious degenerative issues.

Chapter 6

The Gravitational Line

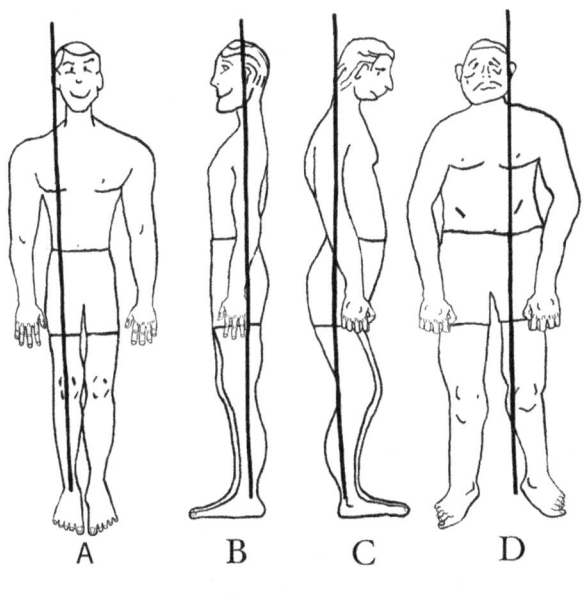

A　　B　　C　　D

Illustration 9

The gravitational line is an invisible force of polarized energy that allows the body to stand erect without effort. When standing, a straight vertical line of energy defines the gravitational line connecting the ear to the shoulder, the shoulder to the hip, the hip to the knee, and the knee to the ankle as seen in the above illustration (B).

Standing is effortless when one maintains posture within the gravitational line because the muscles that move the body keep perfect tension in space. Each muscle has a partner to keep their relationship of balance intact. If one falls away from this energy line, however, gravity will continually pull the body in the direction it leans. For instance, if one rolls one's shoulders inward, it will fold the upper body forward and out of the line of gravity, thus creating a pulling effect, as seen in illustration 9 (C). When the muscle-balance relationship is challenged, the body will compensate by changing posture to keep the body balanced.

Dr. Hiss cited that the individual involuntarily adopts a bad posture in an effort to minimize pain and thus falls away from the gravitation line (1933).

Efficient and fully functioning feet allow the body to move with greater ease than when the foot has succumbed to weakness. Any part of foot function that is compromised will be felt all the way up the body (i.e., the flexibility of the foot is directly proportionate to the flexibility of the spine and vice versa), and standing and movement will require more effort.

Healthy movements of the feet depend in large part on the capability and potential of thirteen lower leg muscles that attach to the foot. Similar to the mechanics of clockwork, these muscles puppeteer the feet into action and must maintain perfect tension in order to keep the foot functioning optimally.

When one wears a high heel, the relationship of the muscles of the front and back of the body become distressed and no longer have equal strength to keep the feet and body stable. This in turn initiates strain that accumulates throughout the day as the body tries to maintain an upright position while standing on *stilts*.

Chronically raised heels create an imbalance of the long foot muscles that propel and assist in balancing the body while moving, throwing the entire body out of kilter.

The calf muscles, specifically the gastrocnemius and soleus, become very shortened when wearing high heels, and because of their large size and connection to the heel bone, via the Achilles tendon, they will tug at their attachment site. These calf muscles are important propellers of foot movement. The prolonged, shortened position of these muscles makes them bulky, minimizing their potential power to allow the foot to take a healthy stride and disrupting the balance of the shin muscles. The perfect and natural organization of the foot will then begin to weaken and break down, and the beautifully intricate ligament structure that holds the bones together becomes strained, and even torn, by the imposition and assault caused by shoes, maiming the foot into uselessness.

I hope you choose to open your eyes and heart to this important information. I suspect many readers will feel very challenged at the thought of changing their shoe style; this is, however, an invitation to step out of the shoes that have been binding you and your feet and celebrate with a happy dance.

I am confident in saying it will make a tremendous difference in how you feel and will add quality to your life.

(See appendix A for images of feet posture in shoes.)

Chapter 7
What It Means to "Reflex" the Feet

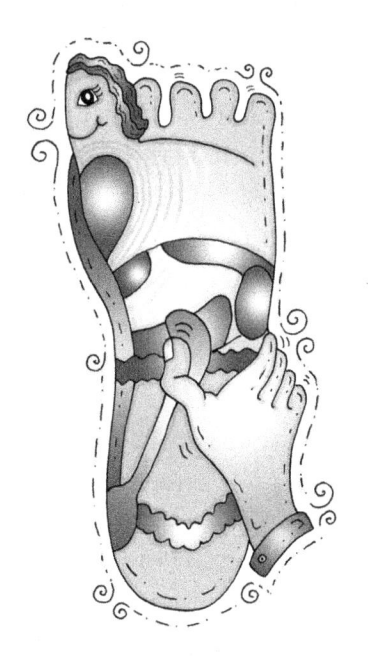

Illustration 10

In research by Christine Issel, and explained in Issel's book *Reflexology: Art, Science & History*, she claimed that beginning 1771 German physiologist Johann August Unzer used the term *reflex* in the neurological study of motor reactions (2014). By 1833

English physiologist Marshall Hall introduced the term *reflex action*. The source behind these terms stemmed from their study of the relationship between stimulating the skin and an internal bodily response.

Through the years pressure has been used as a stimulant for internal healing purposes, and through the practice of trial and error, this guided health practitioners to the feet as a conduit for healing.

As a result of their close and immediate connection to the brain, the feet act very similarly to the brain in that the reflex points in the feet exist as reference points of information to keep track of the vitality or breakdown of the rest of the body.

The reflexologist understands that discoloration or a raised texture on the feet indicates the possibility of a disturbance related to another area of the body. If it manifested systemically from the body to the foot, the affected areas would be organ, blood, and glandular related. If the issues manifested from the foot to the body, it would pertain to the structure and balance of the body and manifest in the skeletal and muscular systems first. If the issue of structure is not corrected in the feet, however, it eventually affects all of the systems.

The feet take on the appearance of each individual body and carry a map of the body's history and current health.

I witnessed one amazing example while I was working as a treatment massage therapist in an osteopathic office. I was treating a patient who suffered with severe neck and back trauma and a brain injury her insurance company was questioning. My job was to provide treatment massage in the trauma areas of the neck and back.

Out of curiosity I asked this patient if I could see her feet, and she allowed me to take a look at them. I almost gasped aloud when I saw both of her great toes appeared swollen, reddish-purple, and warm, and the skin was peeling like an onion. I asked her if she had injured her toes and she said no, that they started to look like this shortly after the accident but they were not painful. The great toes are the reflex areas to the head and brain. As a reflexologist, I considered that her discolored toes indeed expressed injury to her head and brain.

The feet and hands assess our environment and communicate this information to the brain. On a microcosmic level, the brain registers everything happening in the body and marks it on the end of the nerve terminals of the feet. The reflexologist palpates these nerve terminals and will feel a raised texture beneath the skin if there is a matter of which the brain is keeping track. Through various methods of thumb and finger reflexing, the practitioner begins to smooth the raised area to match the texture of the skin around it. The brain constantly assimilates what it is feeling and relaxes, taking the entire body into account, and responds to this stimulus of touch. This ultimately allows the energetic density of the raised tissue to dissipate and be transformed. Essentially, when we touch the feet, we are touching the brain.

The brain sends off chemical and neuro-muscular signals to the feet to move the body from one place to another. This happens instantly and is something we don't have to think about. When the feet move, they relay information up through the spine to the brain, and the brain responds to the command. This connection is constant, and for this reason, I'm convinced that, although the feet don't take on the appearance of a brain, they act very similar to the brain. The brain, like a computer, will keep track of everything we do and experience in our lives and keep a record in our cellular makeup.

According to Dr. Mary Tuchscherer's study, *An Introduction to Peripheral and Central Reflex Activity: A Means of Understanding Reflexology*, "The feet and hands take up more space in the brain than any other part of the body" (1993). (See illustration 11.) This statement rings true to me. As primary sensory appendages, the feet and hands have nerves connected to the entire body. Dr. Tuchscherer emphasized that stress dominates space in the brain, leaving little room for logical, rational, and creative thought processes. Addressing the nervous system through the feet and hands will help the brain recover from stress quicker, thus creating a more efficient, productive, and calm body.

Illustration 11

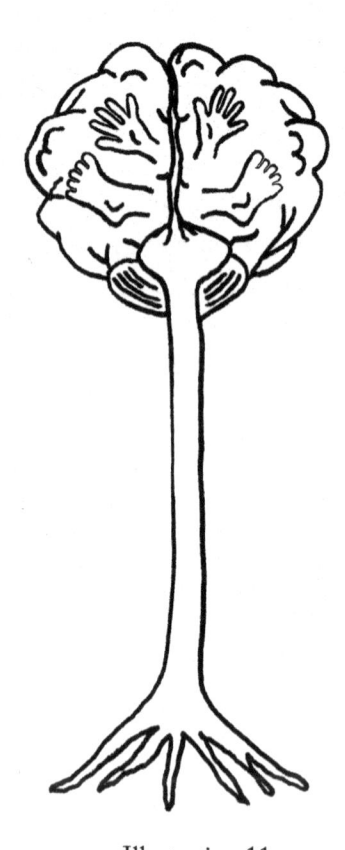

Illustration 11 shows how I envisioned the brain to look with the feet and hands taking up space.

Chapter 8
Theories about Foot Reflexology

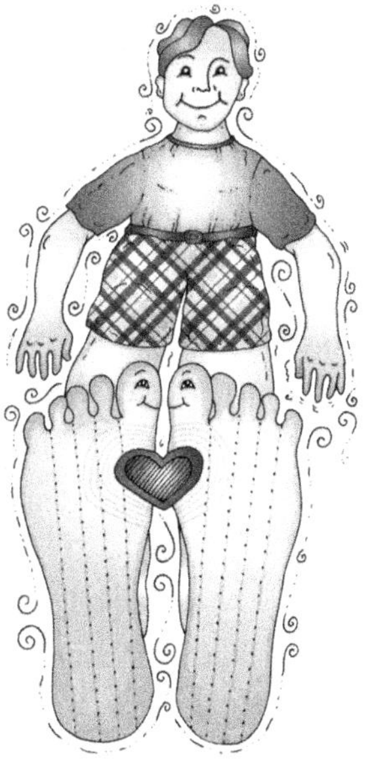

Illustration 12

The Zone Theory

In order to begin understanding how the feet are a mirror image of the body, one must learn the concept of the zones of the feet and body.

In the late 1800s, Dr. William FitzGerald, MD, a University of Vermont Medical School graduate, and his colleague, Dr. Joe Shelby Riley came up with a successful means to administer surgery without pain (anesthesia was not invented at that time). They discovered compressing certain areas on the feet created a numbing effect in a direct line to the body above them. To expand on this insight, they divided the body (head to feet) into a grid of ten vertical lines they coined "zones," using the toes as the dividing lines (1917). This allowed them to explore the feet as a beacon of the body, which allowed them to identify and link specific areas of the feet to other parts of the body by the use of pressure.

Horizontal lines were also drawn on the body and feet to narrow their scope of investigating specific sites on the feet. This helped them to isolate the anesthetizing effects to the affected areas in the rest of the body. With much practice and continuity, it soon became apparent to Dr. Riley that the feet were a microscopic equal to the body above them.

As a result of this finding, they confidently used instruments to apply steady pressure within the zone lines on the feet to create a numbing effect specific to the intended area on the body that needed surgery, which they were able to perform without causing pain to the patient.

They proved this theory, and in the early 1900s over two hundred doctors incorporated zone therapy (1917) into their practice.

Thanks to Eunice Ingham, a physical therapist who worked closely with Dr. Riley, reflexology was introduced outside of a hospital setting, as she devoted her life to training anyone interested in learning this healing art. Rather than using instruments, she taught thumb and finger-walking techniques to stimulate responses in associated parts of the body by using the ten vertical zones as guidelines on the foot to identify the feet more clearly as a microcosm of the body above them.

The Nervous System Theory

According to Café of Life Chiropractic, the average human brain has about 100 billion nerve cells, and there are forty-five miles of nerves in the skin.

These nerves preserve and foster health and vitality by constantly communicating with the body to make alterations necessary for homeostasis.

Reflexing the feet is done with the intent to smooth out neural pathways within the zones to clear imbalanced energy disturbances. The feet act like a motherboard, with over two hundred thousand nerve endings. Any disturbances along neural pathways leave their mark at the ending of nerves in the form of raised texture. The act of reflexing the feet helps to iron out, smooth, and soothe the frazzled ends of the nerves, transmitting a calming effect through these circuits and throughout the body. This soothing effect on the nervous system helps to recharge the body from heel to toes and from foot to head.

We sense our environment with the bottom of our feet and hands to know where we are in space, discover texture, assess for danger, and feel pleasure, to name a few. With this knowledge, it's clear why reflexing and manipulating the feet can create dramatic changes in the body. The comforting touch of graceful hands soothing achy, tired feet is a heavenly experience to the entire body.

Relieving tension or pressure on the nervous system through the feet can soothe the neural sheaths so communication can be transmitted to and from the brain and on to the appropriate channels in the body more directly. A frazzled person will create a rigid neural avenue for communication, and the information pathway will become less efficient and even distorted, confusing signals and messing up the circuits. This is called *stress*. Reflexology is proven to be one of the best tools for dramatically reducing stress because of its calming effect on the nervous system.

My Theory: Efficient Foot Function

Foot reflexology happens naturally during the rhythm of walking and running and in all the ways we use our feet. Advocating for healthy foot function and integrating methods of correcting foot tension that inhibits the foot from optimal function helps to maintain vitality throughout the body.

The majority of my clientele come for relief of various types of foot pain, and all of these clients have been wearing either the wrong size shoe or a shoe style that hinders the foot from moving the way it is designed to move. After assessing the feet and relieving the troublesome muscles and ligaments that have become distorted and injured from constant strain in an ill-fitting shoe, their foot pain is successfully alleviated. Reflexology and massage are applied throughout the session to gauge texture changes in the foot, soothing the tension sites, and soon the compensated posture of the body melts away. The subsequent effects of wearing functional shoes continues to relieve upper body compensation caused from the ill-fitted shoe and rarely gives the client a need to come back again.

Chapter 9
The Controversial Reflexology Map

In 1996 I attended an International Council of Reflexologists conference in British Columbia and was surprised to hear the council president address the subject of eliminating the foot reflexology maps. Her reasoning behind this stemmed from the incongruities of a multitude of foot reflexology maps circulating throughout the world. She thought this made it more difficult for the field of reflexology to be seen as a viable profession.

Although I concurred with her in some ways, it also struck a chord within me. I feared eliminating the map entirely put the field of reflexology at risk of becoming obsolete. Since the practice of reflexology is based on using a rudimentary map replicating the foot as a template of the body, if the foot reflexology map didn't exist, this principle would change.

I spoke up, however, and said, "I heard Deepak Chopra once say, 'You cannot cut into the brain and find the mind.' I believe this is so with the feet. You cannot cut the foot open and see the reflexes, but they are there." The audience stood in ovation with this comment, and I felt relieved that I was not the only one in the room who felt this way.

A foot reflexology map is important because it serves as a tool for understanding where a body's challenges lie. If there are no tension issues in the feet, the feet are relaxed, and so is the body. When the feet, however, present areas of tension, it is a sign that the muscles and ligaments that move the feet are under strain, which impacts how the body moves. The tension produced at the tendon sites on the foot will throw off appropriate weight distribution, creating an inflammatory response in other parts of the body due to the ensuing compensation.

My personal viewpoint of the reflexes of the feet does not stop at the feet but involves taking a three-dimensional mind's-eye journey up and within the body to where compensation resides as a result of foot weakness. When looking at the feet as a perfect match of the body, the trained eye of the reflexologist can detect signs that tell the story of where the body has become stressed.

Adhesions (areas of strain) on specific reflex sites beneath the skin of the foot often confirm an irritation in the corresponding area of the body. These reflexes associated with the rest of the body usually coincide with a muscle that is attached at the same site. It is the tension of the muscle that triggers the reflexive response because of the postural compensation that follows.

Structural Reflexology® is a true science. It's not a mystery once one understands how the complex movement of the feet creates a reaction up the body and out the head. A well-balanced foot will hold and move the body gracefully, whereas feet with misalignment will make the body wiggle and wobble in an effort to find balance.

It takes more than just reflexing the feet to create a lasting change in the compensated body above them. It also takes an astute comprehension of a foot reflexology map that is organized proportionately to the anatomy of the human body, as well as foot anatomy and function, and knowledge of how the dysfunctional foot will manifest havoc in the body above it. It also takes an understanding that shoes have a great potential to limit foot function and may create unbalanced tension in the ligaments that stabilize the bones of the feet and in the muscles that move the feet; this points to how compensation directs the body to fold in and maneuver itself in distorted ways in an effort to maintain balance, posture, and movement.

Over a period of time, the subjugated foot will develop adhesions in the muscles of the lower leg and at their attachment sites on the feet. These muscle and tendon attachment sites, as well as the ligaments that keep the bones of the feet in place, will develop calcium deposits from the strain on the feet. This is what reflexologists feel with their thumb and finger. So they are more than just reflex sites communicating strain in another part of the body; they are also conveying local foot disorder, and this awareness must be considered first and foremost to make a lasting impact on the overall health.

When these adhesions build and persist, the tension will be felt all the way up the body and remain in a specific area where the body is forced into compensated movement and posture. Reflexing adhesions on the feet will relax the tissue, which relaxes the proprioception (the ability of the muscle to know its potential) of the entire muscle and all else within and along the zone. This then frees up the compensatory site. This feels good until you put the shoe on that doesn't fit, and soon the compensation builds again, perhaps creating a different issue next time.

I was recently invited back to be a guest speaker for the *Survivorship Now* Cancer Educational Center. These forums are set up to help survivors find ways to come to terms with their condition and to seek healthful ways to regain their wellbeing and self-empowerment.

The subject I speak on is always related to Structural Reflexology®. The initial response I get when people hear the word *reflexology* comes with skeptical looks from the audience. That is until I speak in terms of the science behind reflexology, and this is accomplished by familiarizing them with the practice of Structural Reflexology®. My students and clients, often in expression of relief, have told me that Structural Reflexology® is what resonates as the truth of how reflexology works.

After viewing and hearing my three-dimensional and personally animated Structural Reflexology® presentation, listeners are more easily able to visualize these ideas. I guide them in building their awareness of how the feet take the body through space by the simple act of walking and how this sets the tone for the way the body responds to this movement.

One of the participants at this forum asked if Structural Reflexology® could help relieve the numbness in her feet. I mentioned that my success with helping relieve numbing in the feet comes from improving the mobility of the joints that stabilize the movement of the foot with the intention of releasing the impingement on the nerves that may be causing the numbness. I also informed her that her numbness could be coming from her low back, in which case the numbness may not be foot-related. I told her we could check the foot reflexes associated with the low back to verify this. She conceded that indeed she did have surgery on her low back with the intention to relieve the numbing in her feet without success and now experienced a lot of low back pain as well.

To emphasize where on the foot she would find the reflexes associated with her low back pain, I directed her attention to the image on the PowerPoint slide, where I placed a side-by-side profile of the vertebral spine and the profile of the arch of the foot. The truth became clear when she realized the painful site she was experiencing on the arch of her foot was specific to the L5, S1 reflex area (see illustration 13), which was associated with the very site of her low back pain.

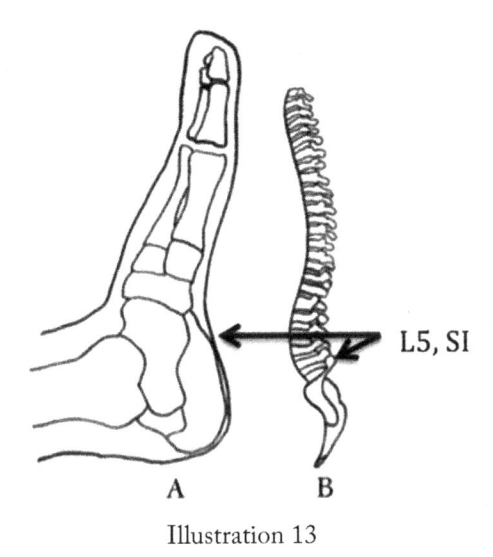

Illustration 13: A is a view of the medial arch of the foot. B shows the curves of the vertebral column matching the arch of the foot.

All eyes and ears perked up at this confirmation. The participants then paired up, and I guided one group at a time in using their thumbs and fingers to examine the arches of their partner's feet. They were directed to search along the arch of each foot for tenderness. Once they found a site of tenderness, they were instructed to use their thumb and fingers to gently ease out the pain while working within the pain-tolerance of the individual.

After exchanging fifteen minutes per participant, they were asked to walk and notice the difference in how they felt. The woman I worked with stood up gingerly, seeming to expect the usual discomfort, and in surprise told me she felt some improvement. In fact, she phoned me the following day and made an appointment while voicing her relief in the numbing of her right foot.

The beauty of reflexology is that it's simple and everyone can benefit. Whether one receives fifteen minutes or an hour and a half, the normal length of time for a thorough Structural Reflexology® session, one typically leaves feeling better.

The feet are the record-keepers of all seen and unseen in the body, including one's emotional wellness. The potential to strive or thrive is truly in our power.

Chapter 10
The Disappearing Little Toe

Illustration 14

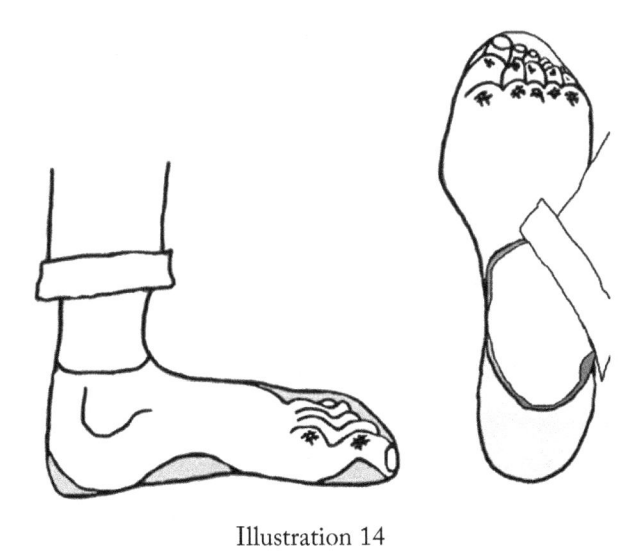

Illustration 14 shows how toes will curl to fit the shoe and become useless from inactivity.

Over the years I have heard teachers and the like mention that evolution will claim the little toe because we don't use it.

Unfortunately, this statement could become a reality—not because of nature, but because of man and our shoe choices. "Use it or lose it" speaks very true to those who choose to stuff and tuck the forefoot into a narrow and tapered shoe.

The toes haven't a chance in the world of functioning this way, and they become deformed and crippled, similar to the effects of foot-binding.

The toes are responsible for keeping the body balanced when striding from one foot to the next, and the broader the stance of the toes, the more relaxed the shoulders and head will be during this transition. The function of the little toes is essential to keep the body balanced to sustain the weight of the shoulder girdle, and any weakness of the toes will be felt in the shoulders, neck, and head. A good mantra would be "strong toes breed strong shoulders and necks." The moment the toes have lost the ability to balance the body, the shoulders have to roll forward and draw in to match the narrow base the shoes impress on the toes. The degree of compensation will be equal to the degree of the narrowness of the toe-box of the shoes.

Inactive toes will cause further issues involving the circulatory processes of the body. Dr. Wikler observed that compensatory posture from weak toes will not only cause the shoulders to roll in, but it will influence the efficiency of lymphatic flow in and out of the axillary (armpits) area, hindering the elimination of waste (1953).

Among many alarming observations about the damage caused by shoes, Dr. Wikler found a very clear link between wearing high-heel, tapered-toe-box shoes and breast cancer. He asserted that the chronically raised heel causes the skeletal position of the shoulders to change its normal alignment, which leaves the ligaments that hold the breast tissue in place vulnerable to irritation. Furthermore, he also stated the postural changes high heels impose upon the pelvic girdle may likely create an unstable environment for the uterus, and cause inflammation of the fundus (top of the uterus), which, according to Dr. Wikler, is the most common site of uterine cancer (1953).

There are so many signs indicating that foot function dictates the physiological balance of the body. When one understands the delicate function of the foot and how it is designed to stabilize and move the body, it seems obvious to side with their preservation. Looking at the feet as a replica of the body above them gives one a looking glass to assess one's own state of health. The power is truly in our hands, or should I say, our *feet*.

Chapter 11
Learning How to Walk Again

Illustration 15

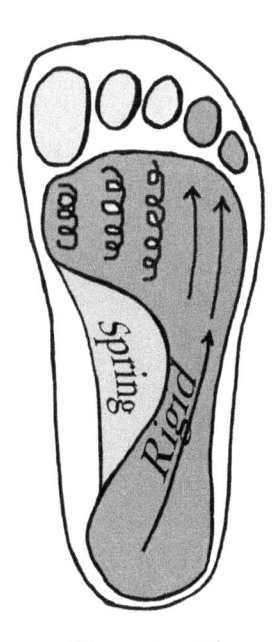

Illustration 15 shows a foot in a shoe that fits. The arrows indicate the path of weight bearing.

In spite of all the walking we do and the fact that the foot has the potential to move in 150 ways, most people take walking for granted. They shuffle on their way, apathetic to the real power of the open stride. For this reason, I feel the need to describe what the body does when we walk.

Momentum of the body begins as the foot lifts from the ground (or steps out) and the heel of the foot touches the ground. Weight is then guided to the outer heel along the outer side of the bottom of the foot. The balancing muscles of the lower leg engage and lift the arch of the foot to encourage weight to the lateral (or outside) side of the foot. When weight reaches the mid-outer foot, the muscles found along the outside of the lower leg counter-balance to prevent the foot from bearing too much weight on that side and contract to direct the movement of weight to the balls of the foot. When the weight is transferred to the forefoot, each toe will bear equal weight in descending order from the fifth to the first toe. The spring-action of the medial arch and the great toe muscles then thrusts the foot off the ground in a moment of balance, preparing the other foot to engage in the same process (Hiss, 1949).

Illustration 16

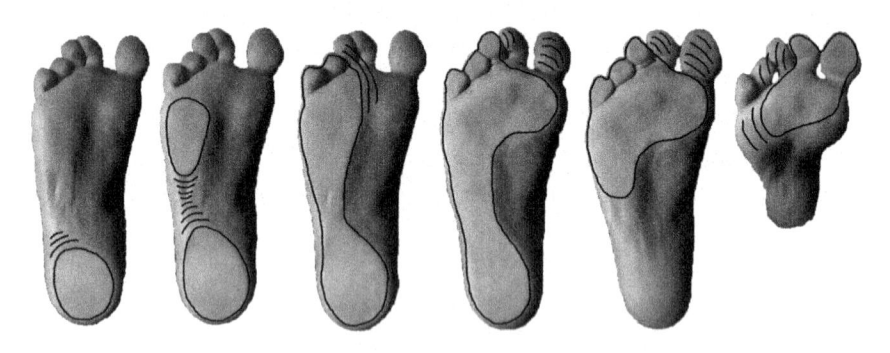

Illustration 16 is an image of the right foot in normal weight-bearing motion. (See appendix D for how this foot movement translates to the reflexes of the body.)

Providing room in a shoe for the toes to wiggle and move is essential to balance the body while the transition of weight is carried from one foot to the other. If a shoe binds the toes, the foot will lose power and potential to propel the body, and thus it minimizes movement to a shortened and less productive stride.

When toes become inactive and unavailable for the final thrust of movement into the next step, normal weight distribution becomes awkward and balance becomes a real issue. Consequently, if the toes are not functional because they are being squeezed into a taper-toed shoe, or a shoe that demands the toes clench to keep it from flying off (such as a flip-flop, clog, rigid cork base, or any shoe that does not have a heel strap to support the back of the heel), the muscles of the neck will contract and stiffen because of the instability of the base. This stiffness in turn inhibits the nourishing and cleansing function of blood and lymph flow specifically to and from the head and brain, causing stagnation of waste, which will almost always present as chronic conditions such as sinus congestion or allergy symptoms and other degenerative challenges.

Illustration 17

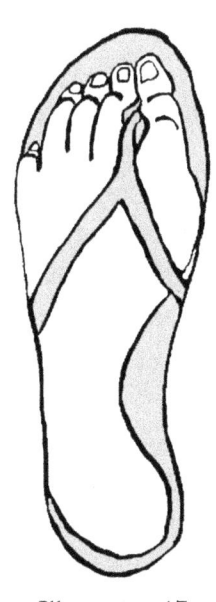

Illustration 17 shows toes clenching the flip-flop to keep it from falling off, which greatly diminishes their ability to stabilize and move the foot.

Quite often my clients have reported a significant decrease in allergic events after wearing functional shoes that allow their toes to relax.

A remarkable change happened with one of my clients who reported that after one session with me, getting into a size-and-a half larger shoe with a wider toe box reduced the tinnitus (ringing in the ears) he had been suffering with for years. This session helped to open the pathways of vitality as his body normalized from chronic compensation.

When congestion persists in the nasal passages, one should examine the style or shape of one's shoes and consider the possibility that cramping one's toes together is causing these symptoms.

A Structural Reflexology® session offers one the option to make informed and wise choices as one transitions back to the natural foot concept. With practical education about how the foot works, this information can be applied immediately and with lasting results. After the session one can walk away enriched with tools one can personally use to facilitate one's own improved health.

I applaud those who purchase minimalistic shoes as opposed to those with rigid soles, as this type of shoe offers the foot a greater range of movement and exercise, which we all know is the key to building strength. It's helpful, however, to learn about how your feet are supposed to work before jumping on the minimalistic bandwagon to avoid harming your feet.

If you are not inclined to go barefoot and have been wearing a rigid-soled shoe, there is a transition period that must take place before one can acclimate comfortably into a minimally soled shoe.

You would injure yourself if you spent twelve hours working out at the gym for the first time. The same rule applies to exercising your feet as you would the rest of your body. True, the feet may feel tired and achy at first when wearing a more flexible shoe, but that is the nature of building any muscle strength. Flexible shoes do not harm the feet and are not to blame for foot pain. The minimalist shoe demands the feet to perform and will expose sites of joint and muscle tension that were brewing from their previous style of shoe. Therefore it is best if they are worn gradually so the feet can relax and ease into a healthier stride; however, they first and foremost must be the correct size for your feet.

People often ask me how reflexology helps those who can't walk. For the paralyzed, reflexology on the feet alone will still be enormously helpful because it's a wonderful way to relax the rest of the body. The soothing effect on the nervous system will promote more efficient blood delivery, which supports improved circulation of the lymph, oxygen, and nutrition to keep the body healthy and vital. During a reflexology session, one of my quadriplegic clients said it best: "I can't feel what you're doing to my feet, but it makes me feel so good." He told me that he especially appreciated how well it helped him release his bowels and that reflexology always left him feeling calm and peaceful.

Chapter 12
Madeline

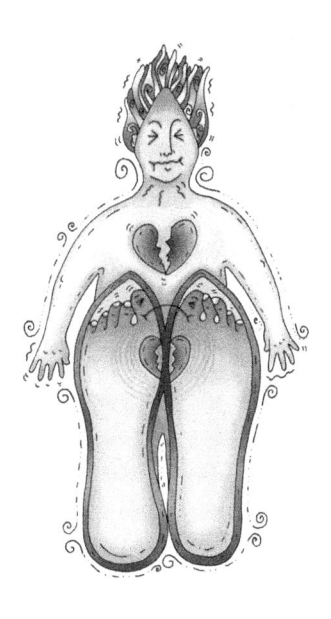

Illustration 18

One of my graduate students asked me to address the topic of bunions in this book. I'll call her Madeline.

Madeline was a participant in one of the many reflexology classes I taught as an elective in a local massage school here in Vermont.

I often began the class by asking willing participants to lie back on the massage table so I could examine their feet, and the other half of the class observed while I guided them through a visual assessment of each individual's constitution based on what I saw on their feet. It was always fun and a great orientation to learning to see the feet as a microcosm of the body.

When I got to Madeline's feet, I saw numerous sites of callusing in very specific areas that were red and flakey. She also had a vertical scar from an incision on top of her left foot that led to her great toe where, she said she had undergone bunionectomy surgery a few years prior. Her right foot had an obvious bunion (a medical term for dislocation of the great toe) that had not undergone surgery and had similar calluses on the bottom of her wide feet.

I could tell she felt somewhat vulnerable exposing her feet to the class as I looked at them with a close eye. She mentioned that her feet were in chronic pain, and based on the shape of her feet, I speculated that her neck and upper thoracic area also had to be presenting challenges, the area between her scapulae must be under chronic strain, and perhaps she was experiencing thyroid issues. I asked if she wore rigid and backless slip-on shoes, as her feet took on this form, which, in my opinion, was weakening her already compromised feet because of the physical and energetic effort it takes to keep this type of shoe on.

On an emotional level, judging by the lateral direction of her great toes, I ventured to ask if she wanted her life to move forward but found that something often sidetracked her. Teary eyed and in amazement, she affirmed all I said was true.

Subsequently, she decided to make an appointment with me to help with her chronic foot pain. I measured her feet to find she was wearing one-and-a-half size smaller than what the Brannock Measuring Device had recommended. My assessment for Madeline's feet was that she suffered from extreme muscle and joint tension in her feet caused by wearing shoes that were too small and a style that inhibits normal foot function.

I was certain this was the cause of her foot pain, her tired legs and hips, her neck and shoulder pain, her daily exhaustion, and her inability to move forward in her life.

How did I know all this without having touched her feet besides measuring? Her feet as a microcosm of her body reflected these answers to me.

The type of shoe Madeline was wearing confused the muscles that move her feet because her toes were too busy holding this backless, rigid shoe in place. It limited her ability to use her feet to walk forward, which necessitated the need to use her hips to lift her foot off the ground. Her toes were strongly involved in clenching the shoe, so they lost their ordinary function. This also forced the feet to splay outward to widen the base of her feet, which made her waddle side-to-side, rather than forward and backward, hence her confusion on how to move forward in life.

In Madeline's case, the larger muscles that move the hips rose to the occasion to move her feet. This, however, is not their job. Eventually the thigh muscles will enlarge with the effort, and the ball and socket joints, in which the hips normally move become weak, which is exactly what happened to Madeline.

In her situation, while wearing this rigid, slip-on shoe, the muscles in her lower leg and foot were not able to function and move her feet and body normally. The muscle tension this caused weakened the ligaments that held her foot bones in place, which then led to foot misalignment.

This shift in foot alignment encouraged inappropriate weight-bearing, causing calluses to form to reinforce the tissue in the areas of the foot that were bearing too much weight.

The talus (the main bone that allows the ankle to hinge and direct weight to the outside of the foot to walk) moved out of place from its position between the lower leg bones and the heel bone. The misaligned talus produced a hyper-pronated condition that torqued the position of the muscles that move and stabilize the great toe. This tension inadvertently moved the first metatarsal and great toe out of place, and voila, a bunion developed. (Which again, is no more than a dislocation to varying degrees of the great toe.)

To help Madeline recover, each session consisted of reflexology, treatment massage on muscles and ligaments under strain throughout the foot, ankle, and lower leg, PNF (proprioceptive, neuromuscular facilitation) stretching, and passive foot mobilization techniques to bring the feet into a comfortable position. I gave her simple and effective daily exercises to strengthen the feet and to help keep them aligned.

Madeline showed improvement with each session and was so excited with her progress she enrolled in my master's of reflexology certification school. While her feet healed, she gained energy, and the red calluses began to fade away.

Today Madeline expressed that her feet feel great, and the pain and callusing have disappeared. Madeline asked me to relay her words that, given her experience, she regrets having the bunionectomy and would not recommend it for most people.

Madeline is now one of my best reflexology graduates, and her life moved forward into a very successful Structural Reflexology® practice of her own.

Chapter 13
Columns of the Foot

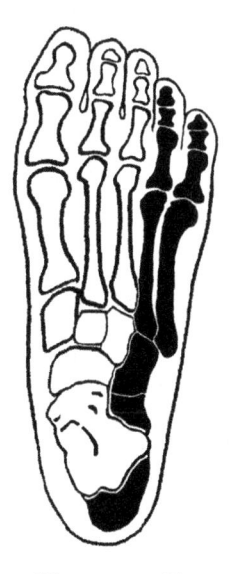

Illustration 19

We are born with over 300 bones in the body, and by the time we reach adulthood we have 206. Each foot has 26 bones and together the feet make up one-quarter of all the bones in our body.

A very important aspect of the anatomy of the foot is its division into two columns.

These two separate columns of bones in each foot have independent functions (see illustration 19). The function of the outer (lateral) column of shaded bones, consisting of the calcaneus, the cuboid, fourth and fifth metatarsals, and the phalanges above them, is to bear and transfer weight when walking.

The medial column, which sits just above the heel bone, consists of the talus, navicular, cuneiforms, first, second, and third metatarsals, and phalanges above them. The function of the medial column is to spring and absorb weight while the foot is being propelled.

Lateral Column	Medial Column
Calcaneus	Talus
Cuboid	Navicular
Metatarsals 4 and 5	Cuneiforms 1, 2, 3
Digits 4 and 5	Metatarsals 1, 2, 3
	Digits 1 2 3

This becomes a very important factor when shoe shopping, because you want to choose a shoe design that will accommodate and encourage both of these functions. However, most shoes are not designed with function in mind, and because of this the columns of the foot lose their independent purposes, undermining their potential to provide functional and efficient movement. The flexible shoe will offer the foot more range of motion, and in turn it will strengthen the foot, creating a flowing, unencumbered gait.

The feet, weighing only 2 percent of our total body weight, are capable of 150 different movements if they are well-aligned and free to move. The flexibility of a shoe determines how much the foot is allowed to access these movements. The stiff shoe will, at best, allow one or two laborious movements in one plane (flexion and extension) at the ankle and some of the toe joints. Just like a building would topple if the foundation were built too rigidly, the feet become wobbly when they are unable to adapt to postural changes in a stiff shoe,

Put Your Best Feet Forward

causing the body to compensate and struggle to maintain balance and comfort in movement. Throughout the day this compensation will build on itself and throw the body out of its gravitational line, creating exhaustion with even the most menial of activities.

Fatigued muscles become powered by deoxygenated blood, which produces lactic acid, and soon one is burdened with muscular pain throughout the body. Too tired to provide their normal levering, the muscles become distorted by this compensation and start to tug on the bones to which they are attached, thus creating subluxations along the spine and feet, and unable to prevent it from happening, one adopts a bad posture. (See illustration 20C &D.)

Illustration 20

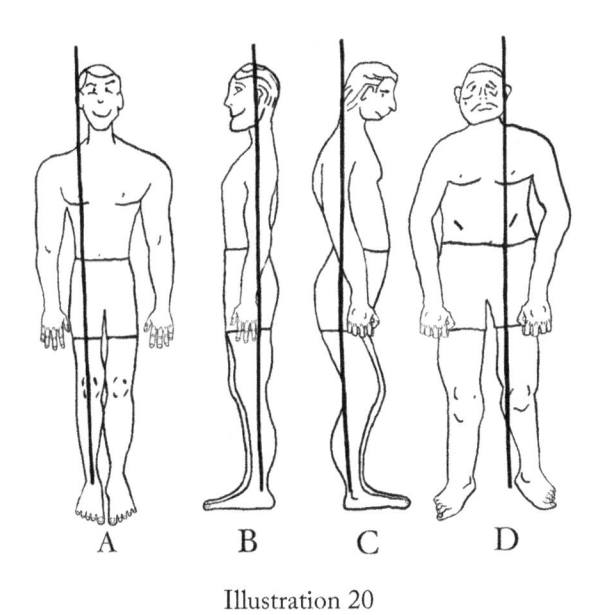

Illustration 20 A and B shows the line of gravity in which the body must align to maintain a comfortable posture. Images C and D show the posture of the body out of this gravitational line.

The bare foot functions on all the planes on which the foot is designed to move and is ultimately the best way to keep your feet and body strong, vital, and happy.

A prime example of structural misalignment of bones in the lateral column of the foot is the scenario that occurs if the joints that stabilize the cuboid bone become locked. The hip and knee will be directly affected because they depend on the foundational function and stability of the cuboid bone to direct movement gracefully.

The cuboid bone is considered the keystone of the foot and needs to be completely stable to perform its job while weight is transferred from the lateral column of the foot to the medial column of the foot. A cuboid bone out of commission means it will not be able to bear weight, so weight will default to the medial column, or arch of the foot, prematurely creating a hyper-pronated condition, or what is commonly referred to as a "fallen arch."

The more appropriate term to use here is "broken arch," which speaks more to structural challenges in the arch's functional integrity and to the misplacement of the bones that make up the transverse arch, not to an age-related phenomenon.

The transverse arch acts as a horizontal bridge to direct weight from the lateral column of the foot to the medial column. During locomotion, as weight is received by the cuboid on the lateral column of the foot, it initiates the other bones of the transverse arch on the medial column to spring and absorb weight rather than to bear weight.

When any one of the bones of the transverse arch become locked or displaced, weight bearing becomes distorted and/or the arch collapses. Dysfunction of the transverse arch becomes evident by the strain and fatigue in the muscles that move the arch, causing them to splint.

The propelling muscles of the foot (the calf and toe muscles) get confused by the dis-orchestration of the mal-aligned foot, alter their function, and shorten and curl under the strain. Miraculously, these long muscles that attach to the foot can keep up this circus act for years until they become so overwhelmed with fatigue that foot function becomes nearly impossible, leaving most people confused as to how this came about.

The opposite can happen when shoes that are too small torque the foot into hyper-supination. Bowing the foot up, and too much to the outward side of the foot affects the position of the calcaneal bone, and turns the heel inward (signs of this point to the well-worn outer heel of the shoe). This arrangement makes the management of weight difficult, and to those afflicted, it will feel like walking with the brakes on.

The long lateral foot muscles that encourage weight toward the metatarsals and toes become fatigued by the long stay of weight on the lateral column of the foot. This imposes strain and fatigue on the muscles of the outer leg that in turn render the foot unable to direct weight toward the metatarsals and toes with ease.

The muscles that move the hips and the ligaments that keep the pelvic girdle stable will also become disorganized under the strain of the medially rotated heel. This traveling tension continues to moves up the side body, causing the shoulders to roll inward, matching the degree of the medially rolled-in heel, which in turn reduces the capacity of the diaphragm muscle to move air in and out of the lungs.

Chapter 14

The Cinderella Stepsister Complex: Understanding the Silent Breakdown of the Foot

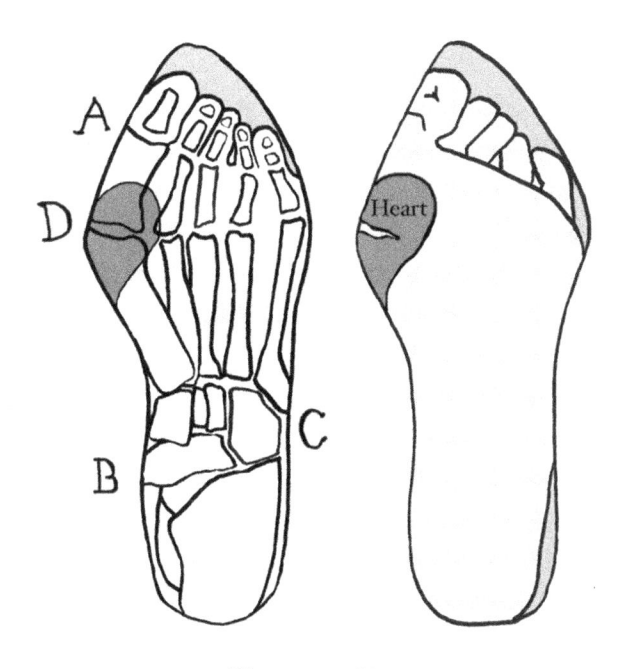

Illustration 21

I'm amazed at how often I hear people say, "I'm breaking in my new shoes" as if it is normal. This is difficult for me to fathom because it perpetuates the idea that the foot should be forced into a shoe that obviously doesn't fit, creating an image similar to Cinderella's stepsisters insisting on making the glass slipper fit. The truth underlying this concept is the shoe is breaking the foot.

We are all guilty of walking around the shoe store convincing ourselves that the shoe will work once it gets stretched out enough. But in the back of our minds, we sense that something isn't quite right. When finding the shoe that fits, there is no break-in period. The shoe should be comfortable the moment you put it on without question.

The image under this chapter title, illustration 21, is a foot in a shoe with misaligned bones labeled A, B, C, and D, which illustrate how the foot begins to break down. Some of the physiological consequences of wearing this shoe are described below.

A shows the toes bound in the shoe. Wearing a shoe with a narrow toe box will create balance issues. One of the most important functions of the toes is to provide balance not only for proper foot function but also to support the heavy weight of the neck, head, and shoulders. When the toes are not available to spread and equally receive weight during locomotion, the upper body becomes vulnerable and responds with intense muscle guarding to help balance the body because the tapered toes are too narrow to carry the load above them.

The wide toe box that fits the shape of the foot will allow the shoulders to remain relaxed, broad, and upright, because the toes will confidently perform their job of providing a stable base while keeping the springing function of the arch and great toe intact.

The area labeled B speaks to pressure and interference in the function of the arch.

Rigid shoes may compress against the delicate muscle tissue of the arch that is designed to provide a cushion for the vital nerves and blood supply that enters the feet at this site. Arch supports also immobilize the arch from its spring and shock-absorbing functions and keep the foot in chronic supination. This confuses the balancing and propelling muscles that move the foot. Thus it under-exercises the muscles that attach to the arch, which overstrains the outer foot muscles and interrupts their part in keeping the foot balanced.

C addresses the cuboid bone, a transition point where the momentum of weight is transferred from the outer mid-foot (supination) and slightly medially toward the toes (pronation).

Success of this movement is based on the stability of the position of the cuboid bone and the cuneiforms, which make up the bones of the transverse arch. (See illustration 22.) The structure of the body depends on the stable function of site C (the cuboid bone) or else the knees and hips will become vulnerable to collapse from the absence of a strong lateral foot base. This is not very productive for the body or the brain that tries to figure out how to move the body without harm.

Any interruption of the function of the transverse arch will make movement awkward and ineffective. This breakdown confuses the balancing muscles that activate the transverse arch mechanism to naturally supinate and pronate the feet while walking, and it ultimately maims the foot into a hyper-pronation.

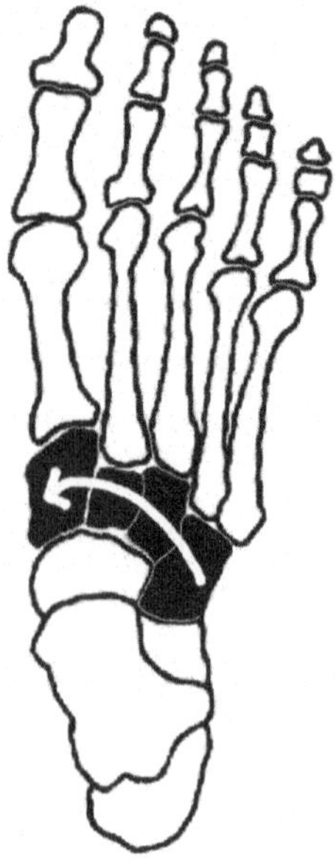

Illustration 22

Illustration 22 shows the front view of the bones that make up the transverse arch and the direction of movement initiated by the cuboid bone.

Though meant to provide support, rigid arch inserts obstruct the crucial steadiness and function of this key transition point of weight transfer by preventing the arch from moving. When the foot loses its shock absorber, the power of movement becomes undermined in its ability to spring and give stability for the great toe to move the body forward. The interrupted flow of weight bearing puts excessive strain on the metatarsals, toes, and great toe, leaving some of the toes without a job and others overworked, especially in a shoe that squeezes the toes together.

D shows how shoes with a narrow toe box force the great and small toes out of place, producing a great toe dislocation (bunion) or a small toe dislocation (a bunionette).

Over a period of time, the strain on the muscles that keep the great toe and small toe in straight alignment will cause those muscles to weaken and create an unstable foot. Unable to adapt to this abnormal toe arrangement, the ligaments holding the transverse arch in place then become compromised, lose their strength, and will no longer be able to keep the bones from moving against the strain. When the transverse arch becomes disorganized by strain, it can no longer direct weight appropriately and one or more of these bones collapse under the pressure of weight.

The narrow, pointed shoe renders the foot incapable of engaging the muscle of the great toe to spring the foot forward, and movement will be defaulted in the direction the great toe is pointing. In many cases the dislocation becomes so severe the great toe loses its function, completely forcing weight on the ball beneath the great toe. Without the ability to spring, and in an effort to protect against this abnormal weight, a callus will develop on the ball of the foot to reinforce and protect the skin and joint. This precarious arrangement will upset the organization of the transverse arch's function to supinate and pronate the foot and cause many other foot disturbances, such as plantar fasciitis, Morton's neuroma, and tendonitis conditions, to name a few.

So the moral is, to avoid dislocations and deformity, choose a shoe that fits the shape of your foot, and whenever possible go barefoot to keep the feet strong.

Chapter 15

Flat Foot or "Fallen Arch?"

It is of the utmost importance to understand that arches of the feet do not fall. This belief that the arch can "fall" has given rise to defeatism (or shall I say "de-feet-ism") surrounding the power of the feet. The mentality that the muscles of the feet naturally become weak with age, and therefore must be propped up, is preposterous.

The long and short muscles of the foot maintain balance and move the foot but do not hold up the arch. Tight leg muscles are the product of weakened ligament issues in the feet and are not the primary reason for foot problems. According to Dr. Hiss, the ligaments of the feet are responsible for supporting body weight and have the strength to carry 7,860 pounds per square inch and have 9 percent stretch and 91 percent elasticity (1933). This is one reason why the feet are so adaptable to the abuse inflicted on them by shoes and can endure thoughtless stress for years without complaint—until they can't anymore.

Props may be necessary for those who have suffered from a debilitating injury such as an impalement, amputation, or osteotomy, or to those with loose ligament structure caused by severe trauma to the foot. As for the majority of the public, however, foot issues can be helped with a little knowledge and the correct shoe size. Propping the arch of the foot should only be used very sparingly, if at all, to offset foot pain during the rehabilitation process and not as a permanent appendage for the foot.

The flat foot is not an obstacle with which we need to contend. On the contrary, the flat foot is a foot fully intact with correct alignment and function and should never be propped because of its flat appearance.

The flat foot has every opportunity to be as comfortable as any other foot, and rarely develops foot pain, unlike the higher arched foot. The difference in flat feet and other feet is in their anatomy and how they function. The flat foot does not bear weight the same way other feet do.

In his book *Functional Foot Disorders* (1949), Dr. Hiss said flat feet develop during the early walking stages of life. Due to circumstances of being overweight or malnourished, the soft bones of the feet, which are mostly cartilage, have not become strong enough to hold the weight above them and deform and flatten before the longitudinal arch develops.

He also attributed flat feet to a younger sibling competing with an older sibling by walking too soon, and again, as a result of this the muscles that form the arch of the foot underdevelop and cannot spring the foot into a normal stride. Therefore, the bones develop in such a way that these individuals learn to walk by bearing weight on both the outside (lateral) and inside (medial) of the foot at the same time. The lateral (cuboid bone) and medial (navicular bone) side of the foot touch the ground before movement is directed toward the toes, which is completely contrary to normal foot movement.

The appearance of the flat foot should not be confused with a foot that has misplaced bones, causing the foot to hyper-pronate. The hyper-pronated foot makes the arch of the foot appear flat to the untrained eye because weight bearing has defaulted to the medial column of the foot. Additionally, the hyper-pronated foot appears to have an arch when not bearing weight, and the flat foot appears flat without a noticeable arch, weight bearing or not.

Often, and only detectable by an x-ray, the flat foot has a pronounced protrusion of bone on the arch of the foot (called an accessory navicular) which allows this foot to bear weight comfortably on the medial side of the foot. The functional difference between them is the true flat foot does not exhibit pain while bearing weight on the medial column of the foot, and because of bone misalignment, the hyper-pronated foot does.

All types of feet can develop foot disorders. Structural Reflexology® sessions are useful for correction whenever the foot has lost its ability to adapt when walking or running, or when the bones of the feet begin to lock at specific joints, causing pain with movement, regardless of how they appear.

Children and Bare Feet

Images of a four-week-old fetus in the womb show the fingers and toes developing on the body wall, and at six weeks the hands and feet become flattened to form the hand plates and footplates before any other organ has taken shape (Sadler, 2010). For this reason, I strongly believe the brain, feet, and hands are inseparable.

Illustration 23

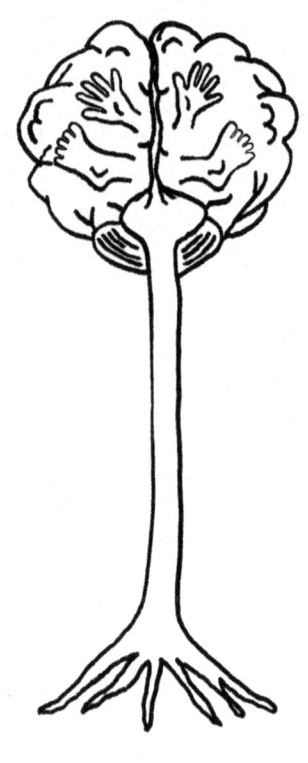

Illustration 23 is an image of the brain, with the feet and hands within it, and the spinal cord.

The bones of a baby's feet are made up of soft cartilage and can be easily disfigured by shoes and socks that bind the feet.

Crawling helps the baby's foot muscles strengthen, and as the muscles get stronger, the baby will decide to walk. With each walking attempt, the bones of the baby's foot will become stronger and begin to ossify enough to bear the weight of standing. Just because they can stand doesn't mean you need to put shoes on their feet to help this process. This would only be a disservice to the child who is learning to develop balance in the feet alone. Always keep in mind their bones are still soft and impressionable to shoes. Babies who walk barefoot will have a better chance developing a stronger core, leaner muscle mass, and broad shoulders to match the proportion of their base (i.e. their shoulders won't roll in because the little toes haven't been scrunched in shoes).

If a child wears shoes before the age of four, the shoes will rob the child of learning to let the feet carry them without the influence of shoes. At this age, shoes will impact the development, shape, and function of the foot and force them to walk in a way that may not be natural to them, and their body will develop while compensation forms their posture.

Dr. Wikler emphasized if you must put shoes on a baby's feet, they should be no more than a protective covering, such as a moccasin style (completely flexible) that is a little wider in the forefoot, more secure in the heel, and that ties or fastens with Velcro onto the foot. Leather is best because its composition is compatible with our skin (1961).

When choosing a shoe, ask yourself, "Would I put these shoes on the baby's hands for hours on end?" Imagine how debilitating this would be for their fingers. Soft gloves or mittens would still allow function, but they would also protect and allow movement. This concept should be applied to the feet as well. The more flexible the shoe, the stronger and more capable the foot will be into adulthood.

A baby's metabolism runs very high, and this produces heat, so unless the baby's feet and hands are cold to the touch, keep them barefoot! In *Take Off Your Shoes and Walk*, Dr. Wikler wrote: "Children who regularly go barefoot, develop stronger, healthier and more functional feet" (1961).

As the baby grows, forty-five bones are formed in each foot. By the time he or she reaches adulthood, he or she will have twenty-six bones, plus two or more sesamoid bones.

Although an x-ray may define the bones in a child's foot, it will not show how soft and cartilaginous they are. Based on the following illustration of postnatal bone development, one can clearly see how impressionable the tissue of a child's foot can be to deforming shoes and socks, causing people to question their belief that their deformed toes were because they were "born that way."

Based on foot development, there are many times when deformity can manifest, and yet our feet manage to overcome many obstacles. Isn't it time to give thought to what we do to our feet?

In illustration 24 of postnatal development of the foot, notice that the heel-bone (calcaneus) appears six months after birth, followed by the development of the talus one month later.

The metatarsals develop in the seventh week of life as well as the tip of the toe, but the rest of the toe bones between them haven't even taken form yet. These bones eventually develop in stages over a period of eighteen years before they fuse together.

Put Your Best Feet Forward

Postnatal Development of the Foot

Epiphysis appears 10th year until puberty

Calcaneus
6 Months

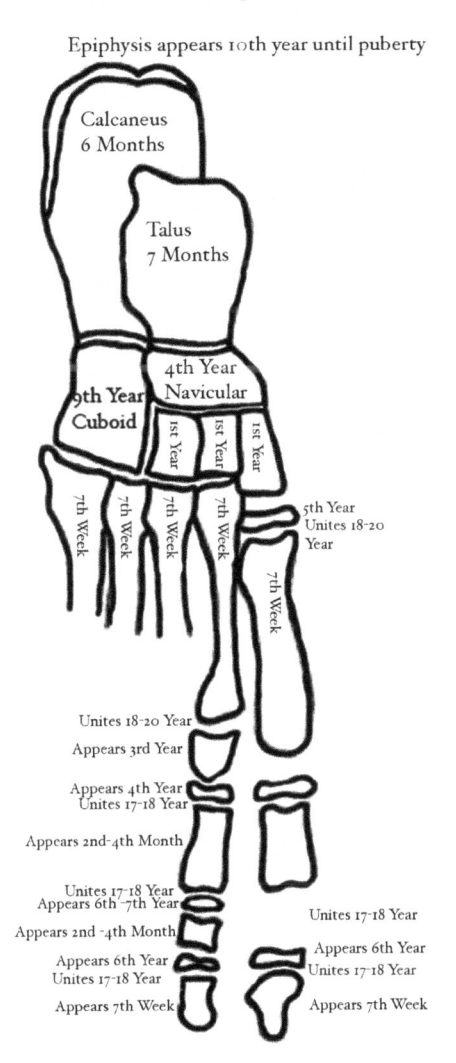

Talus
7 Months

5th Year
Cuboid

4th Year
Navicular

1st Year

7th Week

5th Year
Unites 18-20 Year

Unites 18-20 Year
Appears 3rd Year

Appears 4th Year
Unites 17-18 Year

Appears 2nd-4th Month

Unites 17-18 Year
Appears 6th-7th Year

Appears 2nd-4th Month

Appears 6th Year
Unites 17-18 Year

Unites 17-18 Year

Appears 6th Year
Unites 17-18 Year

Appears 7th Week

Appears 7th Week

Illustration 24

Chapter 16
The Nature of the Foot

The adult foot is made up of twenty-six bones with two or more sesamoid bones held together by 107 ligaments and a multitude of connective tissues. The movement of the foot comes from seventeen lower leg and foot muscles, thirteen of which originate around the knee and attach to specific sites on the foot.

Each muscle that moves the foot has its own function in lifting and placing and propelling the foot to accommodate for weight distribution and locomotion. The thirty-eight joints in each foot provide balance and articulation in order to keep the body sturdy. The ankle is a hinge joint comprised of the lower leg bones (tibia and fibula), the talus, and the calcaneus. This joint allows the foot to hinge up and down, and its stability aids in keeping the great toe pointing straight.

The anatomy of the foot is a phenomenal work of art and is designed to provide 150 ways of movement, perfect precision with each step. The accuracy of the aligned foot frees the body to demonstrate greatness. If people were made aware of the power and intelligence of the foot, they would treat this part of the body with absolute respect and love. One should consider the care of the feet as a wise present and future-health investment because the crippling ramifications of not doing so will eventually interfere with the quality of life.

In 1905, Dr. Phil Hoffman, MD, performed a comparative study of the feet of barefoot and shoe-wearing people. The barefoot subjects he chose were from Philippine Malays and Central and South Africa, the shoe-wearing subjects were African American and Caucasian, and the sandal-wearers were from Northern Japan. As *Conclusions Drawn from a Comparative Study of the Feet of Barefooted and Shoe-wearing Peoples* stated,

> The shape of the foot and its range of voluntary and passive motion are practically the same in barefooted and shoe-wearing races up to the time of the use of footwear that compresses and splints the foot, usually about the end of the first year, after which, in shoe-wearers, there is progressive narrowing of the anterior portion of the foot and diminution in the range of motion of its phalangeal, tarsal and ankle joints.

He also concluded that the barefoot subjects' toes pointed straight forward while standing and when walking, or in a resting posture, as shown in the following Photos 2 and 3.

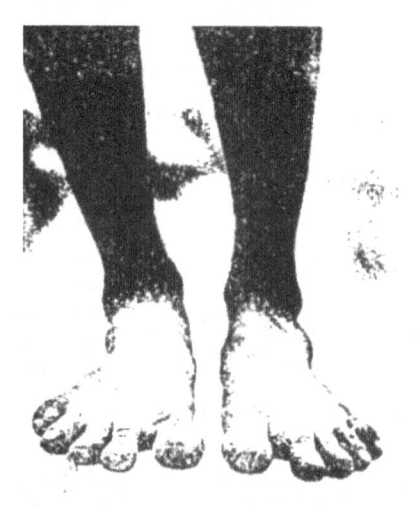

Photo 2

From the *Journal of Orthopedic Surgery*, Volume III, Number 2, October 1905.

Photo 2: Photo two is a dorsal view of weight bearing. Notice the toe separation and adduction of the great toe.

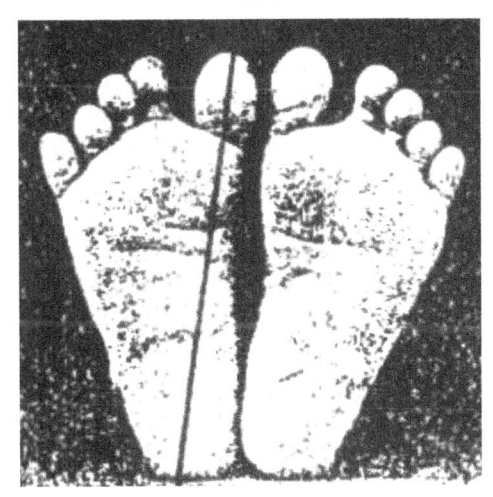

Photo 3

From the *Journal of Orthopedic Surgery*, Volume III, Number 2, October 1905.

Photo 3: Photo three shows the plantar view of the feet with straight and separated toes. Notice the widest part of the foot is at the toes.

In this study, Dr. Hoffman observed that the shoe-wearer's feet were everted (toes pointed outward), both in a standing position and with movement (see Photo 4). The shoe-wearing subjects' longitudinal arch had weakened, as did the ligaments of the feet and the leg muscles that control foot movement. The "longitudinal arch" Dr. Hoffman speaks of is also known as the arch of the foot.

Geraldine Villeneuve

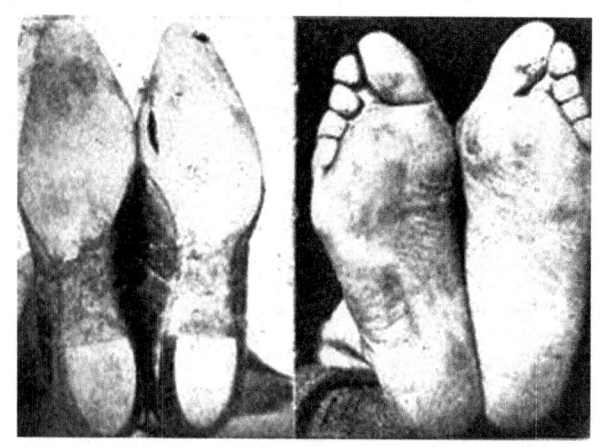

Photo 4

From the *Journal of Orthopedic Surgery*, Volume III, Number 2, October 1905.

Photo 4 shows a predominant type of footwear and its inevitable effect on how the shape of the foot conforms to that of the shoe.

Dr. Hoffman also observed the sandal-wearers' arches showed a bowing of the longitudinal arch, and they assumed a pigeon-toed posture while standing and walking. (See Photo 5)

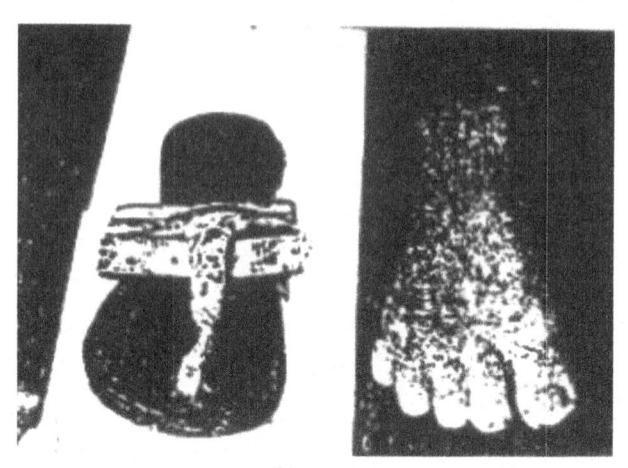

Photo 5

From the *Journal of Orthopedic Surgery*, Volume III, Number 2, October 1905.

Put Your Best Feet Forward

Photo 5 is a photograph of a thong-type sandal and the foot that wore it.

In this same study, Dr. Hoffman traced the feet of nine-to twelve-year-old, barefooted children before and after they wore shoes for almost three months. The astounding results show how shoes can easily compress and deform feet in a very short amount of time, especially at such a young age. (See Photo 6.)

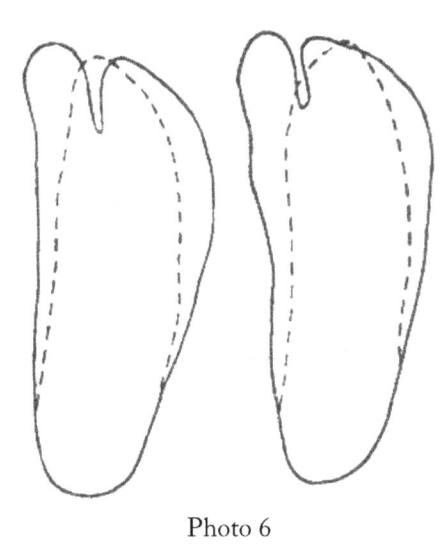

Photo 6

From the *Journal of Orthopedic Surgery*, Volume III, Number 2, October 1905.

Referring to Photo 6, Dr. Hoffman stated,

> This figure represents outlines of feet and their coverings as found in shoe-wearing communities. The solid lines show those of the feet and the dotted ones those of their respective shoes. These are not exceptional but average illustrations, and fairly indicate the pressure to which millions of human feet are subjected day after day through a lifetime. The feet in time become so used to compression that they cease to be conscious of it.

Geraldine Villeneuve

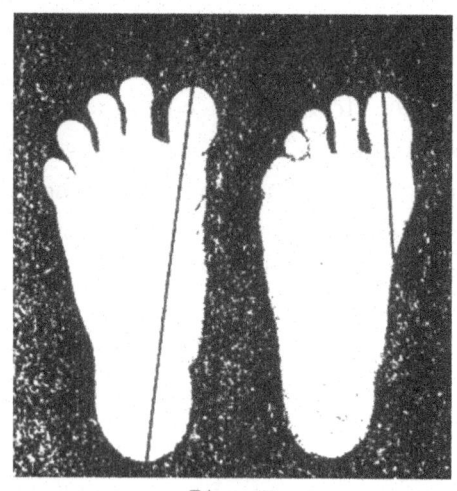

Photo 7

From the *Journal of Orthopedic Surgery*, Volume III, Number 2, October 1905.

Photo 7 above is one of Dr. Hoffman's photos of a before and after image of a child's foot after wearing shoes for three months.

This study revealed how deforming shoes are to the feet, and there is also evidence that shoes can contribute to harmful effects on the body as well.

After treating over ten thousand patients with foot problems, Dr. Wikler reported that there was not only an improvement on the relief of foot pain, but he also noticed symptoms of other health issues presented by these same patients started to resolve on their own. For this reason, he suspected many ailments could be attributed to the misaligned foot. After years of compiling his notes, he confidently deduced that 15 percent of degenerative diseases were linked to shoes. The significance of the study was so alarming to Dr. Wikler he felt strongly that a health warning should be written on specific shoeboxes, as 15 percent was the percentage that warranted a disclaimer on every cigarette box linking their use to lung cancer.

For what shoes would there be a disclaimer? The answer is any shoe that alters the true dynamics of foot function.

Some people don't take their shoes off until they lay down to sleep. I've even heard people say they never go barefoot and take their shoes off at the end of the day only to slip them into another shoe. This is very distressing to me. Keep in mind your feet correspond to your life and they have the potential to invigorate the entire body or stifle it. When our feet hurt, it shows in our faces. So why not treat them with the respect and care they deserve? Our feet contain all the vitality in the entire body. What do your feet look like? How vital do you feel? Is your body taking the form of your shoes?

Chapter 17
Long Foot Muscles and Their Reflex Sites

As mentioned previously, thirteen of the muscles responsible for moving the foot originate at sites above and below the knee and attach at specific sites on the foot to lever the foot into motion. For this reason they are referred to as "long foot muscles," and these lower leg muscles must be considered when assessing foot problems.

Compression against foot muscles caused by shoes minimizes their ability to move the foot. This constant strain eventually causes muscle exhaustion and tendon strain at their point of attachment to the leg and foot, thus slowly diminishing muscle power. Like driving with the brakes on will produce heat and smoke, the impact of chronic muscle inflammation and fatigue due to ungainly movement creates an environment that produces adhesions in the overworked muscle and in the fascia that covers them. Fascia is a translucent layer of moist tissue that covers and connects all muscles in what Tom Myers calls "trains of fascia." Fascia allows the muscles to move fluidly within this casing; when adhesions develop in the muscle, however, the fascia sticks to this trauma site and pulls the entire train of fascia with it (2016).

This is why fascia also plays such an important role in movement. When the balance of these long foot muscles has been challenged over an extended term, it will eventually throw the body off normal muscle movement and pull at the fascia, affecting the entire body. Misinterpretations of symptoms become common when foot tension or deformity is not considered as a possible lead to the onset of pain in other parts of the body due to the resulting compensation.

For the purpose of clarity, I have chosen to address the long foot muscles that are mostly responsible for balancing and propelling the body and describe how the weakening of these muscles, as a result of restrictive footwear, causes foot problems and compensation in the body.

The Large Calf Muscle (Gastrocnemius)

The large calf muscle, referred to as the gastrocnemius, is the strongest muscle of the long foot muscles, and like the soleus muscle, which lies just beneath this, it acts as a foot propeller. The flexing action of the large calf muscle via the Achilles tendon lifts the heel and points the toes downward. This wonderful and powerful muscle has two heads that split and attach to the back of the knee.

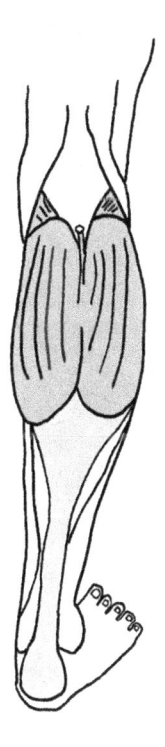

Illustration 25

The large calf muscle (gastrocnemius) as found on the posterior leg.

This large, superficial muscle endures a lot of abuse from shoes, but because of its strength, it retaliates with a vengeance. The first hint of distress on the large calf muscle, after leg cramping, is pain in the heel when placing your foot on the floor. If the issue that causes this pain is not relieved the large calf muscle will continue to contract and pull at the attachment site of the heel bone, causing the ankle bone (talus) to "lock" or shift in its secure position above the calcaneus. The ankle bone acts as a pivotal bone and is held in place only by ligaments. This allows the ankle to hinge and move the foot freely.

When the ankle bone shifts out of its position, it loses its ability to hinge the ankle in its correct plane, which thwarts the alignment of the bones that make up the transverse arch.

Illustration 26

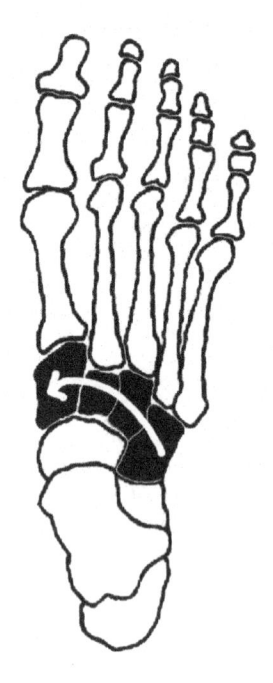

Illustration 26 emphasizes shaded areas on the top of this foot, which are the bones of the transverse arch. From left to right: the medial, intermediate, and lateral cuneiforms, and the cuboid bone.

When the function of the transverse arch is compromised, it upsets the balance necessary for the foot joints to articulate and transfer weight. Consequently, the plantar ligaments begin to strain and become overwhelmed, the fascia becomes inflamed and sticks to the foot muscles, and soon one may be diagnosed with plantar fasciitis.

A common problem that arises from the chronic tension of the large calf muscle is local pain in the arch or heel. Sometimes this can be accompanied by the development of a sesamoid bone in the Achilles tendon that attaches to the heel, known as a "pump bump." Like a kneecap, a sesamoid is an accessory bone the body produces to protect the underlying tissue.

A sesamoid bone can develop in any tendon depending on the need for the body to reinforce the site against excessive pressure and/or weight.

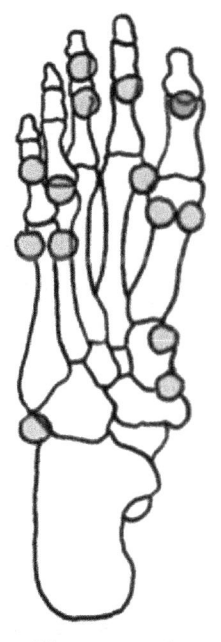

Illustration 27

Illustration 27 is the skeleton of the bottom surface of the foot. The circled areas represent muscle attachment sites where sesamoid bones could develop.

The circled areas in illustration 27 represent sites where sesamoid bones may develop on the bottom of the foot. Normally, an adult will have two sesamoid bones to reinforce weight under the great toe; however, the number of sesamoid bones that appear on the foot will depend on the weight of the individual. An obese person will have more sesamoid bones than a thinner person, who may only have one.

In abnormal circumstances of tendon strain from excessive friction, the body will produce extra tissue to bolster strength at the site and protect the tendon from becoming too frayed. If the situation remains unresolved and the pressure against this tendon is not relieved, the body will continue to produce increasing amounts of tissue that eventually ossifies into what looks like another bone. It often happens to those who wear high heels because of the constant friction against the Achilles tendon; hence, its namesake, the "pump bump."

The "pump bump" may also develop in the back of the heels of long distance runners who run up and downhill wearing rigid shoes. When the arch is propped, it cannot spring the foot into its stride, and the calf muscles (forced to take on this function) become unable to extend with their full potential and become the shock absorber, rather than the propellers of the foot. The brunt impact of the weight irritates the Achilles tendon attachment to the heel bone and develops into a bump of protection to reinforce strength. The longer the irritation persists, the bigger the bump grows. Shoes that are too small may also produce the same condition.

The greatest complaint of excessive tension on the large calf muscle is not so much foot pain as it is low back pain, chronic hamstring injuries, and knee pain. It may also be responsible for inefficient blood flow to and from the heart, lymphedema, and varicosities. (See chapter "Calf Muscles and the Heart.")

The Muscles that Move the Great and Smaller Toes

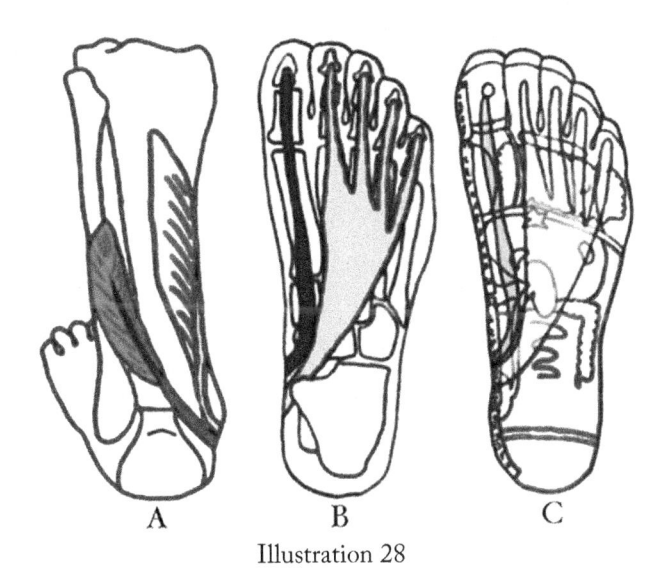

Illustration 28

A: The two muscles in the back of the lower leg that move the great and smaller toes; B: their tendons cross the arch to their attachment on the bottom of the foot to the toes; and C: the reflex sites associated with these muscles.

Most people are unaware that the muscles that move the arch and toes are found deep within the calf muscles.

These long foot muscles are greatly affected by shoes that require the toes to curl to keep it from falling off. This includes any shoe that is a backless slip-on, flip-flop, or a clog style. This may initially sound confusing to those who are accustomed to wearing these shoes because their feet have been clenching the shoe long enough to forget how much energy and focus it takes for the toes to adapt to this demand. Footwear that requires the use of toe muscles to keep the shoe from falling off are a recipe for disaster, and they will eventually breed a multitude of health problems seemingly unrelated to wearing dysfunctional shoes. The biggest perpetrator is the flip-flop.

Illustration 29

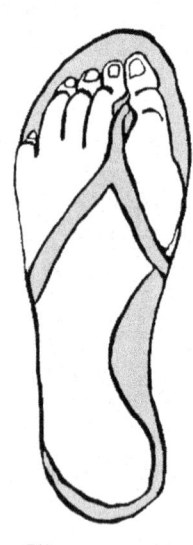

Illustration 29 shows the toes clenching to wear the flip-flop.

Foot conditions and symptoms that tend to manifest as the result of weakened function of the toe muscles include, but are not limited to, hyper-supination of the foot, arch pain, hammertoes, and bunions. The first sign of the development of any one of these problems is noticeable when one begins to default to standing on the outer sides of their feet while standing still. It's the extreme tension of the muscles of the great and small toes that draw the foot into this position, so don't fool yourself into believing this is just a habit that you picked up. The habit is the sign.

The effect of clenching one's toes in a shoe will also make these muscles chronically contract without relief and begin to pull on their attachment to the toes, making them curl into deformity. Shoes that are too narrow and too short are responsible for forcing the toes to curl to fit the shoe. Not only does this shoe create awkward tension in the muscles that move the toes and keep the base of the body stable, but it also predisposes the foot and ankle to chronic sprains and, even worse, avulsion (break) of the bone to which it is attached.

The Main Arch Muscle (Posterior Tibialis)

A   B   C

Illustration 30

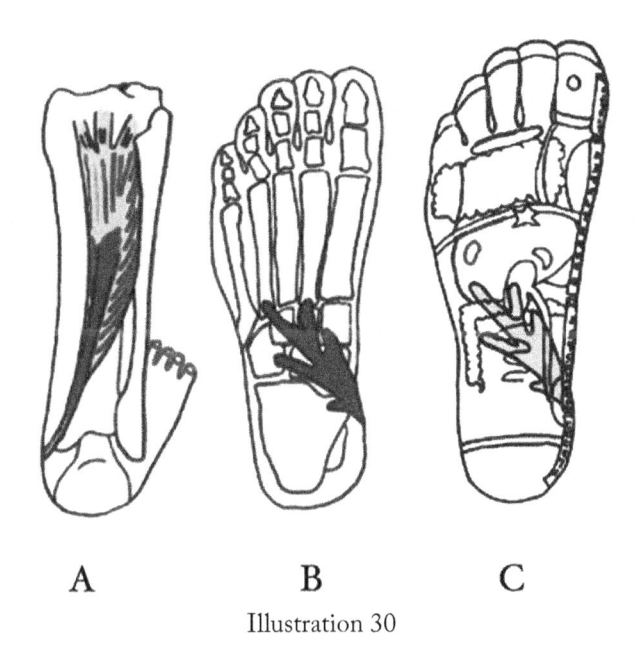

A: The main arch muscle (posterior tibialis) in the back of the lower leg that moves the arch of the foot; B: the tendons cross the arch to their attachments on the bottom of the foot; and C: the reflex sites associated with this muscle.

The main muscle that forms the arch, (posterior tibialis) crosses the arch, and attaches to sites on the bottom of the foot. This muscle originates at the top, outside of the back of the knee beneath the large calf muscles. It is the deepest long foot muscle.

When the main arch muscle is free to extend and contract, it allows the foot to flex downward and inward, and this exercise keeps the arch strong.

The nemesis to exercising the main arch muscle is inhibitors to its function, such as props or rigid shoes. Hard inserts and rigid shoes will prevent this muscle from moving, as it prevents the arch from moving. Balance will become an issue because the main arch muscle (posterior tibialis) will not be able to fulfill its function of keeping weight on the lateral side of the foot during locomotion, and the spring-action of the arch will atrophy and become weak, gradually becoming ineffective as it loses its vitality and strength. Exercising this muscle means allowing the arch to spring without obstructions. In other words, no arch supports.

Typical issues that tend to manifest in the body if this main arch muscle is under strain include back pain (especially low back pain), bladder issues, digestive issues, matters associated with the uterus or prostate, and hip misalignment.

From decades of practice, I have come to the conclusion that all sorts of issues can transpire from wearing shoes that prevent the foot from functioning properly. It could take years, or it could happen overnight. But one thing is for sure: it is difficult to trace problems to shoes if one has no knowledge about how they can affect the feet.

The Long Outer-Calf Muscle (Fibularis Longus)

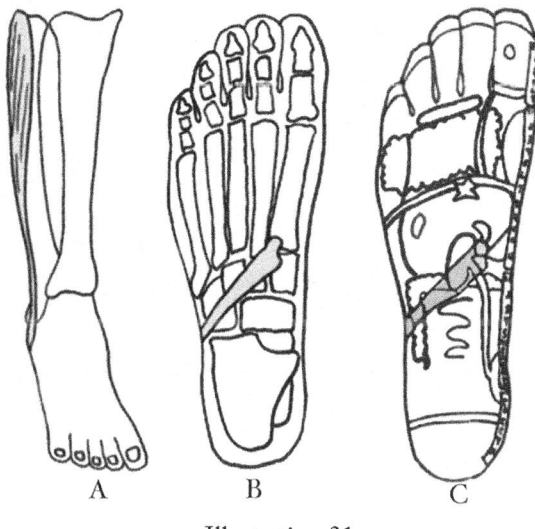

Illustration 31

A: The long outer-calf muscle (fibularis longus) originates on the fibula bone and moves the arch of the foot downward; B: it slips under the foot and attaches to the bottom of the foot under the arch; and C: the reflex sites associated with this muscle.

One would not expect the muscle that runs along the outer side of the lower leg, the fibularis longus, could cause so much havoc in the foot and body if it becomes overly strained. However, the long outer-calf muscle is often responsible for many disturbances of the foot, including pain in the arch, because this is where it is attached.

The degree of eversion, or how far the feet point outward, will indicate the degree of strain to the long outer-calf muscle.

The long outer-calf muscle's origin is on the head and upper two-thirds of the fibula, and it attaches to the arch of the foot (at the medial cuneiform and first metatarsal). Shoes that do not fit the size or shape of the foot will make this muscle bow under tension and pull on the arch of the foot so much that it draws the forefoot outward.

The chronically stressed long outer-calf muscle may first present as pain on the inside of the knee and/or arch of the foot before the pulling effect throws foot mechanics out of balance. If strain of this muscle is not alleviated, the pull at its attachment to the arch can wrench the bones out of place, disrupting the alignment where the first metatarsal meets the great toe.

The muscles designed to keep the great toe straight become challenged with this toppling effect against it and eventually succumb to fatigue. Under this great strain from the pulling tension of the long outer-calf muscle, the great toe dislocates from its position on the first metatarsal, causing the metatarsal head to move inward (toward the midline of the body), and the great toe bone outward, and soon one is diagnosed with a bunion. (See illustration 32.)

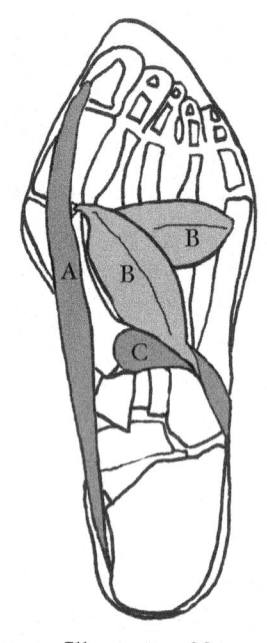

Illustration 32

Narrow toe-box shoes cause tension on the muscles that keep the great toe straight and move the bones out of alignment; A. *Ab*ductor Hallucis; B. *Ad*ductor Hallucis; C. Fibularis Longus (long outer-calf muscle) attachment to the base of the first metatarsal.

Dislocated bones in the feet make the muscles of the feet exhausted and will thwart normal weight-bearing and make movement awkward. This situation compounds over time, weakening the ligaments of the transverse arch, and one or more of these bones become misaligned and throw the foot into hyper-pronation.

Some of the areas affected by excessive strain of the long outer-calf muscle include pain in the knee and hip, as well as low-back pain. This can also cause issues of the thyroid and adrenals, as well as intestinal annoyances.

The Short Outer-Calf Muscle (Fibularis Brevis)

The shorter lateral leg muscle (fibularis brevis) is also a balancing muscle that works with the shin muscle (tibialis anterior) and engages during the transfer of weight from the cuboid, guiding the weight of the body slightly medially and in the direction of the toes. Its attachment at the base of the fifth metatarsal keeps the movement of weight balanced and intact unless the short outer-calf muscle, disrupted from excessive tension, has to constantly autocorrect to keep the body from falling sideways.

A   B   C

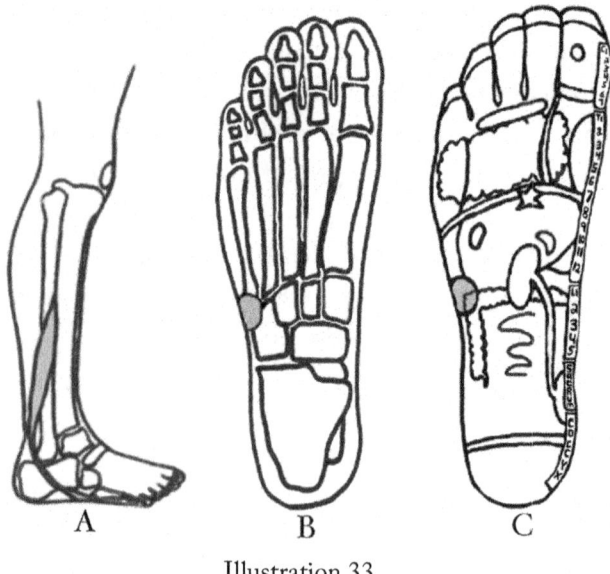

Illustration 33

A: the short outer-calf muscle (fibularis brevis) moves the arch of the foot downward; B: its tendon attaches to the base of the fifth metatarsal on the bottom of the foot; and C: the reflex site associated with this muscle.

This accumulated tension on the short outer-calf muscle is often the cause of the most commonly broken bone in the foot: the base of the fifth metatarsal. Wearing shoes that are too small and narrow for the feet puts severe tension on the short outer-calf muscle. An awkward step on the smallest pebble can instigate the already overly strained muscle to respond in a fast, karate-like defense to keep the body upright. It overcorrects so rapidly that the force pulls the bone off at its attachment site. This is called an avulsion. In other words, it's a condition similar to the straw that broke the camel's back.

When the balancing function of an overly tight short outer-leg muscle becomes impaired, disturbances in other parts of the body will begin to manifest because of compensation. Some of these conditions include chronic sprains in the foot and ankles, hip joint bursitis, and sciatica, and because it attaches at the reflex site of the transverse colon, constipation, as well as other intestinal annoyances.

The Shin Muscle (Tibialis Anterior)

The shin muscle (tibialis anterior) works with the main arch muscle (posterior tibialis) and the long outer-calf muscle (fibularis longus) by providing perfect tension on the arch of the foot as weight transitions from the outer foot to the toes. Their shared tendon connection helps to stabilize the midfoot to allow the arch to absorb the weight of the body.

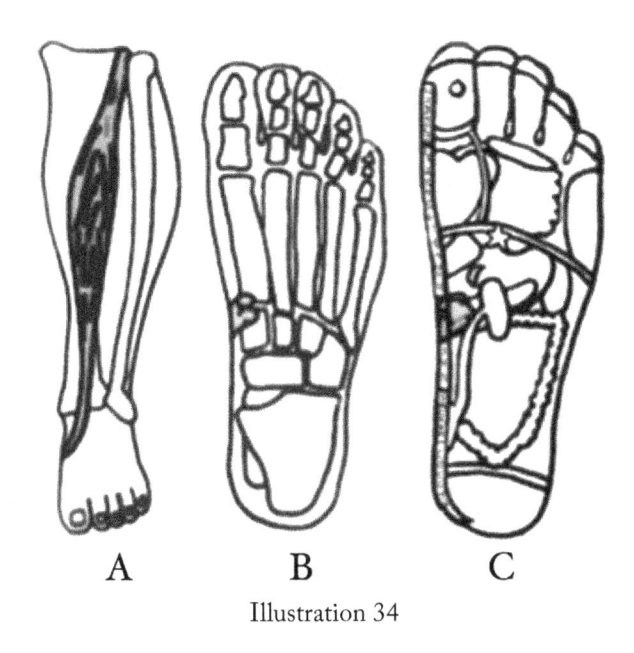

Illustration 34

A: The shin muscle (tibialis anterior) moves the arch of the foot upward; B: its tendon attaches to the arch on the bottom of the foot; and C: the reflex site associated with this muscle.

One knows the shin muscle is under great strain by evidence of shin splints and inflammation due to its lack of movement or from being overworked.

The shin muscle will fatigue greatly if its balancing partners become weak. This happens as a result of joint tension in the bones of the transverse arch, and problems arise in the shin when the arch is propped and immobilized from movement. Props that are placed in the arch of the foot prevent this shock absorber from doing its job, and instead the weight of the body, intended to be received by the strong ligaments of the arch, is abruptly thrust back up the shin bone.

The propped arch puts the shin muscle in a stationary position. Unable to move, it becomes weak from the boomerang effect of body weight being thrust onto it. Overworked and abused, the fascia surrounding this muscle thickens, much like a callus, to protect it from the ensuing chronic inflammation, making recovery of this muscle more difficult.

Incidentally, the consequence of propping the arch on a regular basis is that they will weaken the ligament structure of the foot and make the bones vulnerable to collapse, which contradicts their purpose.

The shin muscle will also become weak if one of the bones of the transverse arch becomes displaced, causing the foot to hyper-pronate. This happens when all the muscles that move the arch stiffen in a show of strength and splint in an effort to prevent the arch of the foot from bearing weight, which is a compensating reaction to protect the ligament structure of the foot. The splinting action of these muscles prevents them from their normal function, which is to move the foot, not to stabilize it, and they become overworked and fatigued, and eventually fail from keeping weight on the outer side of the foot when, finally, the arch collapses.

Typical issues that manifest in the body when the shin muscle is under chronic strain are shin splints, pancreas issues, midback fatigue and/or pain, inefficient pyloric sphincter function (where the stomach contents empty into the small intestines), and reduced range of motion in the low back and hips.

The Great Toe Lifter
(Extensor Hallucis Longus)

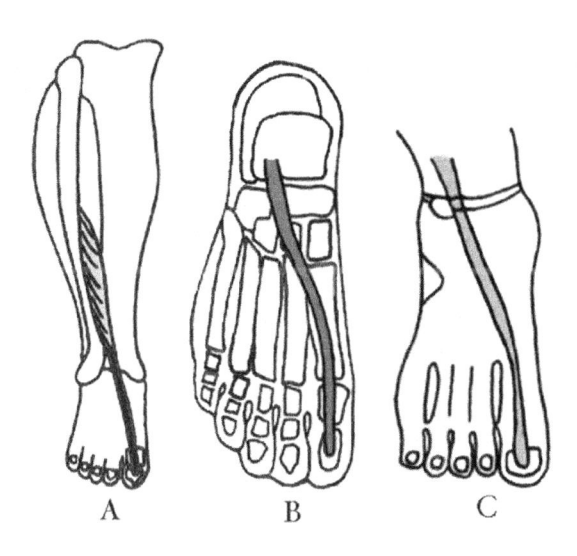

Illustration 35

A: This muscle in the front of the lower leg lifts the great toe; B: its tendon crosses the ankle and attaches at the end of the great toe on top of the foot; and C: the reflex sites associated with this muscle.

The great toe lifter (extensor hallucis longus) plays an important role in lifting the great toe to prepare for the next step. If this muscle becomes weakened from misuse, one will tend to trip a lot or stub one's great toe. Its origin begins on the front lower leg, and it is held in place by ligaments, called retinacula, as it crosses the ankle and attaches at the end of the great toe.

Shoes that require the great toe to incessantly flex downward to keep the shoe from falling off weaken the great toe lifter and will cause it to underperform when the need comes to extend the great toe back. When toe extension becomes laborious, it produces excessive heat, creating an inflammatory response. Over a period of time, the great toe joint, metatarsal phalangeal joint (MPJ), becomes larger in appearance with every inflammatory response, leaving behind calcified waste products in the joint and eventually causing it to buckle or claw.

When shoe shopping, one should consider the muscular effort it requires from any of the toes to keep a shoe from flying off the foot. Some shoes even have a lip that encourages the toes to press against it. This style of shoe would certainly weaken the toe extensors and diminish the lifting and spring capability of the great toe.

Aside from joint buckling, also known as hallux rigidous, and fungal issues of the nail, the chronic strain and imbalance of this great toe muscle extender may contribute to other conditions in the body, such as groin-related tightness and other deep anterior pelvic muscle strain, neck, throat, and thyroid issues, cervical and lumbar spinal misalignment, muscular strain of the muscles along the spine that connect the back of the neck to the pelvis (erector spinae), iliopsoas muscle tension, and jaw strain.

Chapter 18
The Calf Muscles and the Heart

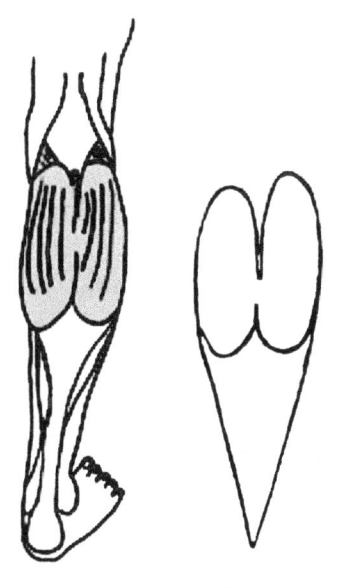

Illustration 36

I recently took part in a 5k walk to support heart health awareness. During my walk, I found myself observing the shoes and gait of some of the participants. I started thinking about information Dr. Wikler shared about walking and running in shoes that don't fit and its effect on the heart muscle. He expressed his deep concern about the dangers of encouraging walking, especially rigorous walking, as a prevention or remedy for heart health without first measuring the feet and advocating for functional shoe wear.

His reasoning came from years of experience and observation that led him to strongly believe many degenerative heart diseases are caused by shoes that are too small. The calf muscles, primarily the gastrocnemius and the soleus, are the largest muscles of the lower leg and attach to the foot via the Achilles tendon at the back of the heel. These strong, propelling muscles allow the foot to extend and contract with movement. Although all the lower leg muscles play an essential, synchronistic roll in movement, the pumping action of the two largest calf muscles (gastrocnemius and soleus) is a specific contributor to the return of de-oxygenated blood back to the heart, and they therefore can be linked directly to heart function.

Because of my experience with clients whose calf muscles become rigidly locked, and who also suffer from poor heart health, it leads me to wonder about the connection between these muscles and the heart.

If a shoe is too small, it will greatly reduce the ability of the calf muscles to extend and contract the foot, and the body will compensate by recruiting other large muscles, such as the thigh and hip muscles, to move the body. The extreme tension that builds in a muscle that is bound in a shoe will create chronic muscle tears and fatigue, creating broader, weaker calf muscles rather than those that are longer and stronger.

As I've said before, walking under these intense muscle conditions would be similar to driving with the brakes on, and the leg muscles themselves would begin to constrict and squeeze the arteries and veins enough to hinder the efficiency of blood flow to the feet and from the feet back to the heart. This muscle pressure against the veins could minimize blood flow enough to keep stagnant waste in the body longer, which oxidizes the body tissue more quickly and could potentially cause a plethora of other degenerative issues because the heart has to pump harder to work against this lower leg stagnation.

Supple calf muscles give the feet more range and leverage to move than shorter, bulkier, calf muscles. (See illustration 37.) Increasing their range of extension and contraction allows them to be a more powerful pump in the action necessary to assist the veins in the efficient return of deoxygenated blood back to the heart. The pumping action of the supple calf muscles also allows the lymph fluid to filter and cleanse the blood to be able to send the collected waste products to the appropriate channels for elimination.

A   B

Illustration 37

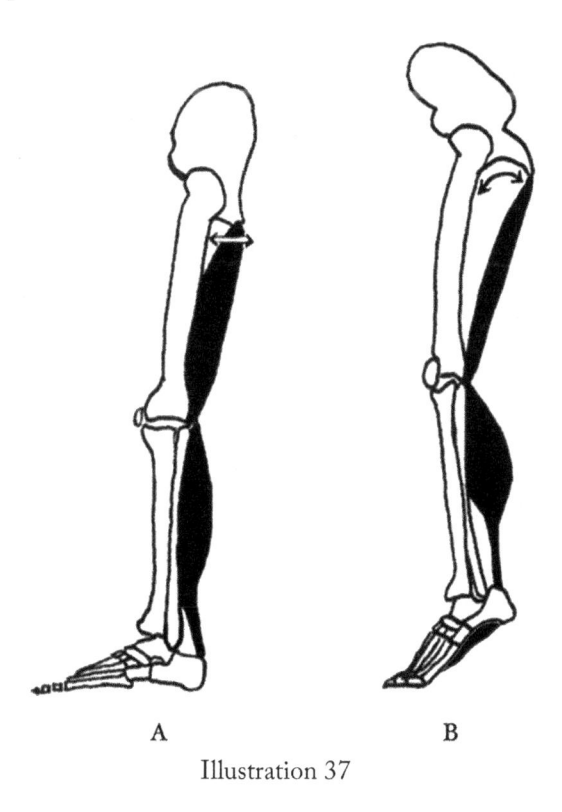

Illustration 37 shows the side of the leg with hamstring muscles as they attach from the pelvis to the back of the knee, and the calf muscles from the back of the knee to the heel. Image 37A shows relaxed muscles with the pelvis in alignment. Image 37B is a view of the leg as if wearing a high heel. The hamstring muscles that attach from the pelvis to the knee become tight, tipping the pelvis. The calf muscles become bulky and short. While the feet and body can adapt to this posture in short increments of time, the chronic muscle compensation necessary to balance and move the body with a chronically lifted heel is likely to create internal organ and tissue inflammation, especially in the pelvic bowl.

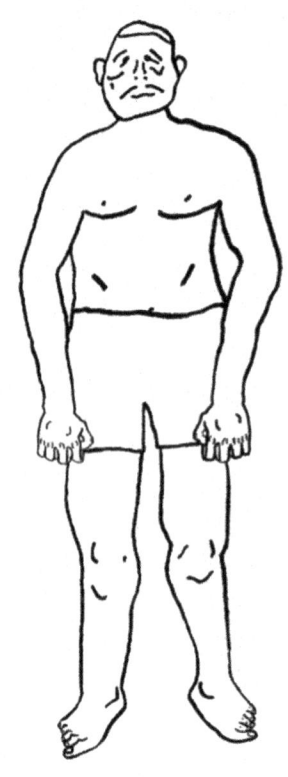

Illustration 38

Another case in point is deduced from illustration 38, which shows compensation due to a misaligned foot. Instead of the toes pointing forward, the foot splays outward in an attempt to make the base of the body wider to help hold the body upright. The everted arrangement of the feet will not allow this individual to propel the body forward in a normal stride and instead will default to waddling side-to-side to move.

Dr. Wikler observed that the postural outward splaying of the feet narrowed the opening of the femoral triangle (found in the groin where the leg bends at the hip), which is the gateway of blood supply to and from the legs.

This deviation gave him great concern for the welfare of the heart because this narrowing could slow blood delivery enough to produce an increase of blood clotting, and therefore rigorous walking or running in shoes that do not fit would only exacerbate a compromised situation. Dr. Wikler was firm in believing cardiac events are often caused by misaligned bones in the feet caused by shoes; therefore, as part of their rehabilitation, he thought it was critical for heart patients to have their feet measured and to receive a full foot assessment before a walking regimen was prescribed to prevent further damage.

Chapter 19

Arch Supports: "'To Be? or Not to Be?' That is the Question"

A few years ago I was invited to be the guest speaker at an annual Chiropractic Association meeting. It made perfect sense to share my insights about foot function and the spine with this respected profession, and honored and thrilled, I accepted. The presentation seemed to be received well until nearly the end of the forum, when someone asked about my thoughts on arch supports. Shortly after voicing my perspective, the mood changed in the room, and I was anxiously and quickly encouraged off the stage. I had hit a nerve.

At the time I was not aware that the main distributors and proponents of arch supports happened to be the audience to which I was speaking. Nevertheless, it is my strong opinion that those who truly need to have their arches propped make up a very small percentage, and that arch-props have been overly prescribed by health practitioners and shoe salespeople without giving enough attention to exploring why one's foot pain occurred. I reservedly understand the temporary use of an arch prop if all other natural foot-alignment options have been exhausted, and I certainly endorse their use in the case that the feet have suffered irreversible damage, or in support of mending a broken bone or an injured ligament.

Over time, however, the use of arch props will propagate structural issues felt primarily in the low back and neck because it immobilizes the function of the spring action of the arch. The placement of a rigid form in the arch of the foot eliminates the waving movement of the arch, which is designed to absorb shock and abruptly reverses the weight of the body back up the body, creating compression in the curves of the spine.

Though meant for good, the long-term use of arch props will weaken the foot further and force it into an unnatural stride, resulting in distorted function of the muscles that move the foot. Furthermore, the abruptness of weight against the arch caused by the prop weakens the ligaments that stabilize the bones that keep the arch strong. This confuses the whole orchestration of the muscles that move the foot, and subsequently the upper body will compensate for the weakening base.

So why not just relax and let the arch support do the work? The answer is, although the prop is doing its job to hold the arch up, it is not correcting the cause of the problem. An arch that is painful is mostly the result of bones being out of place in the transverse arch, or misalignment of the talus. If the arch needs to be propped the cause needs to be found and addressed because in the long run, the arch support will only exacerbate the weakness of the foot, and soon other parts of the body will become equally weakened.

Prevention and education are sure ways to avoid foot problems, and if the problem already exists, there are other ways to correct and strengthen the debilitated arch of the foot without the use of props.

As I mentioned earlier, many well-intentioned health professionals and shoe manufacturers have guided the general population to believe that feet are weak and need to be propped, especially as we age. I find this very disturbing. I have discovered most people are uninformed about how the feet are designed to move and how this movement influences the entire body. The problems the feet are exhibiting are the direct result of the shoes they are wearing. Pain that manifests in the feet is more often than not a symptom of a greater problem happening elsewhere in the foot and is very often overlooked, even by the best health professionals.

It would be unreasonable to expect everyone who wears arch supports to throw them out the window without first truly understanding the mechanics of feet and their vitality, and without finding out why their foot problems developed in the first place. Whether foot pain is the result of trauma inflicted on the feet from an accident or caused from the strain put on them by shoes, there is a certain path that needs to be followed to prepare the feet to be functional again before correction can happen.

First, the feet need to be properly measured. This usually reveals the reason the feet have become problematic. Once shoe size has been determined, the areas of foot joint and muscle tension need to be addressed and relieved for the feet to be comfortable with movement. Once joint tension has been relieved, the feet need to exercise to acclimate to their renewed alignment and to become stronger.

Putting one's feet into flexible shoes without first going through the above stages will often expose the weakened areas of the feet and cause increased pain, so much that it'll be blamed on the functional shoe instead of the shoe that weakened the foot in the first place. The length of time arch supports have been worn will determine the individual's dependency on them and the degree of weakness in the foot and spine.

My compassionate mother called me one evening to say, "A lot of people wear props in the arches of their shoes. Maybe you should be careful about mentioning it in the book." I quickly explained that writing *Put Your Best Feet Forward* is meant to educate the public about why it is so important to build foot strength in order to prevent the need to wear such props. I further explained that arch props in the short term may alleviate the symptoms of foot pain, but in the long term the dependency on them will increase weakness in the feet and will propagate more physical ailments down the line.

I told her *Put Your Best Feet Forward* is about informing others about the health problems that will ensue from wearing rigid shoes or rigid inserts, and that exercising the feet by going barefoot will be the best medicine to regain vitality, power, and health in the feet and body.

A significant number of people suffer from foot pain and have been guided to use arch props as the end-all answer for their pain relief. Most of my clients who enter my office wearing arch supports say shoes were never considered as a contributing factor to their foot pain and their feet were not measured to rule out the cause of the foot problems.

Once the area(s) of joint tension have been addressed the healing begins, follow-ups of rehabilitation help to maintain and build strength back in the foot. This allows the individual to release the need to prop the arch and his or her dependency upon it.

For longevity purposes, it is essential to maintain the integrity, function, and structure of the feet. Unless there is a necessity to mend broken bones, cutting the foot should be avoided. Once the feet have been cut into, there is a great potential for crippling the foot further and causing harm to the entire body.

The common link to this epidemic of foot problems always comes back to shoes, so where does the fault lie? Can you blame the shoe industry for trying to sell shoes? No. Educating the public about the vitality of the feet and the great importance the feet have in keeping the entire body healthy needs to become a common practice, so people can at least can make an informed decision when buying shoes. It's a choice people make, much like the choice one makes to smoke cigarettes. Nowadays, however, there are warning labels on cigarette packages regarding the dangers of smoking.

So I invite you to remember that the feet are more than capable of carrying the body through life, and when the foot becomes challenged, an arch prop should only be used as a very temporary crutch until alignment is possible.

Chapter 20

Common Foot Problems Revealed

If you notice any of the following signs and symptoms, you may be developing a foot problem:

- Redness in specific areas of the feet after taking shoes off
- Blisters from walking with shoes on
- Calluses
- Corns
- Achy, tired legs and feet
- Sweaty, smelly feet
- Fungal nails
- Cramps in the calves and feet
- Knee or hip pain
- Low back pain
- Upper back pain
- Neck pain
- Jaw pain

These signs and symptoms begin with minor warning signals and gradually progress into annoying complaints seemingly far from a developing foot problem. The initial signal of redness caused by the friction of a shoe that doesn't fit is the first clue. With no reprieve, the redness blisters and then calluses. Calluses become inflamed as friction from the shoe pushes against the skin and creates a corn. Continued pressure and tension at the site changes the balancing relationship (agonist and antagonist) of keeping equal muscle tension where they attach, and one overpowers the other and begins to move the bone in the dominant direction. Soon the organization of the foot becomes compromised, throwing off the balance of the body above it. The body responds by compensating because balance becomes an issue. Once the individual reaches this point of foot incapacitation, it is difficult to trace the point of onset, and the initial signal of redness becomes a faded memory, leaving shoes innocent.

Shoes do create most of the foot problems we experience, and heel spur syndrome is often the springboard for the initiation of other foot problems caused by shoes.

Heel Spur Syndrome

Heel spur syndrome is commonly recognized as symptoms of pain in the heel when putting the foot on the floor upon waking.

This condition is often the cause of excessively tight calf muscles, specifically the gastrocnemius and soleus. With little room in the shoe to extend and contract, these muscles bulk up and tug at their attachment and tip the back of the heel upward, putting strain on the bottom (plantar) surface of the foot.

In this case the abnormal position of the heel makes the fat pad move from its protective site where it provides a cushion for the bone spur, the site where the plantar ligament, muscles, and fascia attach. When the fat pad is no longer protecting the site of the bone spur, it and the plantar tissue of the foot become vulnerable to damage, and pain signals the body to produce calcium to build protection at the spur until the pulling tension at the heel is relieved and thus, allows the heel to rest in its natural position. Once corrected the pain resolves, as does the built-up calcium.

Even though, in some cases, x-rays reveal an avulsion of the spur, making one think walking on this bone is why one has pain, according to Dr. Hiss the pain one feels at the heel does not usually come from walking on the spur, but from the discomfort of walking on an excessively tight plantar tendon. The danger of this is that one could be led to believe cutting the spur out would correct the problem (1949).

Measuring the feet almost always tells why the foot is in trouble, and if it isn't an issue in shoe-size, it's the style of shoe that is causing the problem. After the matter that created the problem has been revealed, the structure of the foot is assessed for muscle imbalances and ligament tension. Bulky calf muscles and pump bumps provide the practitioner with an idea of the amount of tension produced at the heel.

Illustration 39

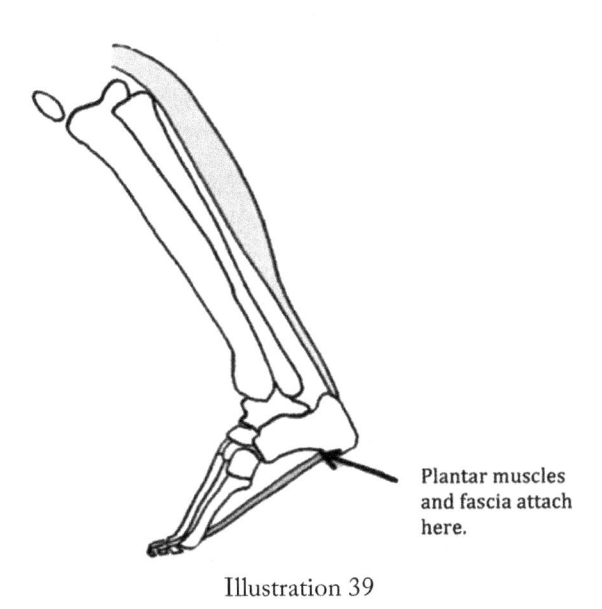

Illustration 39 shows the site of a bone spur, which is also a natural attachment site for plantar muscles and connective tissue.

To relieve this tension, the muscles of the lower leg and foot must be relaxed through various methods of massage. Foot reflexology is integrated into the session to create the soothing effect necessary for the nervous system to relax, which stimulates an improvement in blood flow throughout the body, allowing muscle tension to melt away in the feet and body above them.

The relief of tension in muscles and ligaments of the foot and lower legs also provides relief from postural compensations as foot organization is restored and the heel rests easily on the floor without pain.

While an x-ray can expose sites of foot trauma, it usually does not reveal joint tension or slight bone dislocations, which throw the foot off balance. And if it does, the diagnosis is *arthritis*, passing this condition off as a disease needing management without a cure. Do not despair, however, as most arthritic conditions are joint tension that can be relieved. X-rays will not explain why symptoms of foot pain occurred, and unfortunately the follow-up is often a referral to a surgeon for removal or shaving of the traumatized site when, in actuality, the trauma is often a symptom of tension brewing elsewhere in the foot. That area is usually a misaligned talus or cuboid bone. This explains why bunions and neuromas in the feet often recur after surgery, because the *symptom* was removed, not the cause.

Plantar Fasciitis

Arch pain (plantar fasciitis) often starts with chronic heel pain and then builds into pain in the arch of the foot. This condition is often the result of a misaligned talus. (See illustration 40.) The pulling tension of the calf muscles where they attach to the calcaneus via the Achilles tendon creates an unstable arrangement for the talus and calcaneal connection.

Illustration 40

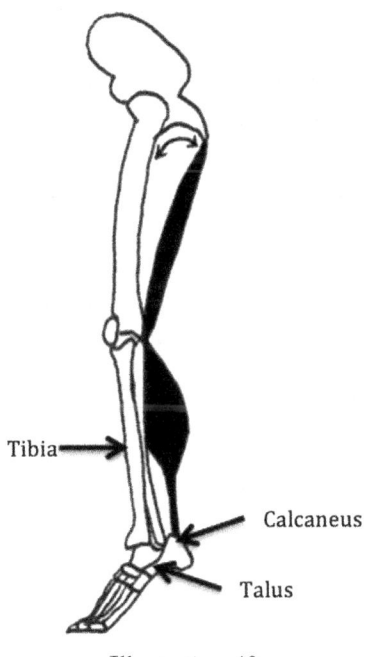

Illustration 40 shows the pulling power of muscles on their attachment to the foot and pelvis. The talus, which rests below the tibia, will become unstable with this chronically lifted position.

The tipped calcaneal bone creates space for the talus to move out of alignment, and thus causes the infamous "fallen arch."

Please be clear that it is the result of shoes that cause the misaligned talus that leads to arch pain, especially high heels, flip flops, and backless slip-ons.

Morton's Neuroma

Morton's neuroma is created by a nerve-impingement in the foot. Symptoms of this condition are commonly described as sharp, burning pain on the top or bottom of the foot mostly between the fourth and fifth metatarsals. Though this syndrome sounds like a dreadful disease, it is mostly a nuisance, and the cause can be easily remedied. The onset starts from a disturbance in the organization of the joints holding the bones of the foot in place, specifically those surrounding the cuboid bone. (See illustration 41.)

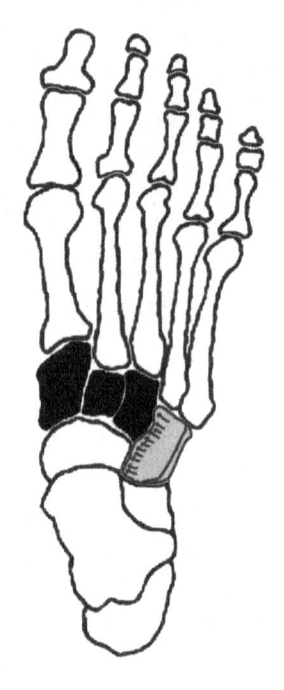

Illustration 41

Illustration 41 is a view from the top of the foot. The lighter area is an image of the misaligned cuboid, which is in a downward and medial position.

The nerve that supplies sensation to the fourth and fifth toes becomes a problematic area when the cuboid bone becomes misaligned. The downward, medial rotation of the misaligned cuboid bone compresses the lateral plantar nerve. The nerve responds by sending sharp, burning pain to these toes, and without relief from this compression, the nerve becomes starved and the toes become numb.

Illustration 42

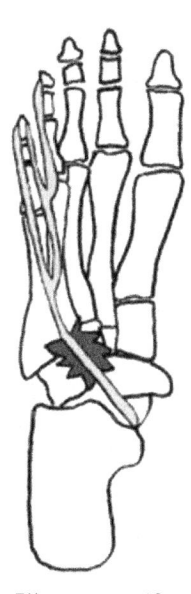

Illustration 42 shows the lateral plantar nerve on the bottom of the foot. The darkened, jagged image is the site of the downward and medial position of the cuboid bone impingement causing symptoms of Morton's neuroma.

The production of calcium around the nerve shows up on an x-ray image and is diagnosed as Morton's neuroma, but do not be alarmed. The neuroma is an internal callus formed around the nerve sheath. To preserve the vitality and life of the nerve, the body envelops the nerve with calcium to create space to separate the bones compressing it.

The genesis of the neuroma is the initial impingement that happens due to complications in muscles and ligament function when feet are bound in shoes that do not fit.

The wonderful news is this condition is correctable without surgery. Surgery will cut out the symptom (the neuroma) without correcting the compression that caused it, leaving scar tissue, and often permanent numbing, in its place. Unfortunately, many of my new clients who opted for neuroma surgery tell me they have another one growing in the same place not long after they had the previous one removed. This verifies that the symptom was cut without addressing the problem that caused it. Cuboid alignment is the way to go for pain relief, and once this manual correction is made, healing can occur as the need for the callus disappears.

The Bunion

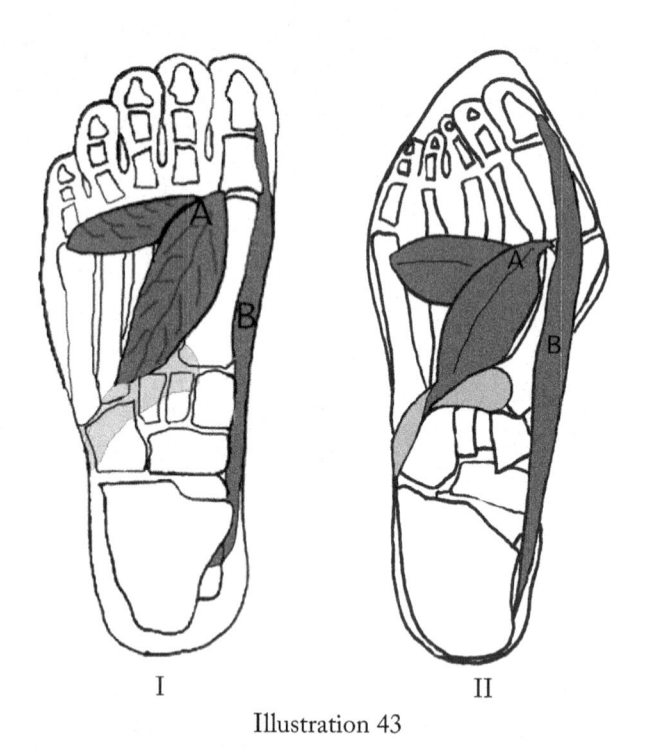

I II

Illustration 43

Image 1 is the foot bones in alignment. Adductor 1A and abductor 1B keep the great toe straight. Image 2 is the same foot with a severely dislocated great toe; adductor 2A and abductor 2B struggle to keep the great toe straight.

When the initial signs of redness, blisters, calluses, and corns are not taken seriously, the next progression in this line of symptoms is joint tension that causes the bone to move out of place to make room for the shoe—in other words, a bunion.

I would consider the bunion as the worst scenario in the breakdown of the foot.

Contrary to what many believe, the bunion is not an inherited condition. The more likely inheritance is the walking pattern one adopted when learning to walk just like Mom, Dad, or Grandma. I saw this happen firsthand when I casually observed my one-and-a-half-year-old niece mimicking her grandmother walking down the hallway in her house.

My mother-in-law has severe bunions and can no longer "toe-off" from her great toes. She therefore has a waddling gait. My niece studied this very adeptly, copied her movement, and waddled down the hall behind her. At first I thought this was cute and funny until I realized this is the moment when the pattern continues.

The bunion (hallux valgus) is no more than a misalignment of the great toe to varying degrees. The muscles that stabilize the great toe become strained in the shoe. These culpable shoes encompass a large range of styles that fall short of truly benefiting the foot in any way, shape, or form. The point is, vitality and power become lost in the leg and foot muscles that are designed to keep the great toe straight and become weak by the strain and effort imposed on them by the shoe design.

The progression of a bunion happens when one or more bones in the transverse arch become misaligned and cause weight to fall on the arch of the foot. This chronically hyper-pronated position encourages the potential development of all the foot issues mentioned above, and if kept this way long enough the muscle that keeps the great toe and first metatarsal straight will weaken and be pulled away from its post, making the first metatarsal bend away from where it meets the great toe.

The possibility of the bunion being inherited could possibly be explained by an inherited arch discrepancy. For example, Mom and Grandma had the same longer arch type as you, leaving you all subject to shoes that are not designed to fit both the length of the foot and the arch size. I strongly believe the strain put on the arch when fitted into a shoe that does not accommodate its arch length is the basis for the developing bunion, releasing the myth that their bunion grew because their mom had one.

To clarify once more, a bunion may develop due to the discrepancy of the arch measurement, as 70 percent of people have a longer arch and 10 percent have a short arch than their toe-to-heel measurement. (See illustration 44C and A.) Neither of these arch lengths meets the design of the manufactured shoe.

To elaborate on the pitfalls of the manufactured shoe, a size 7 shoe is designed with a size 7 arch, and most people have a longer arch than their toe-to-heel measurement; therefore, their arch is too long for the shoe design to rest comfortably. This will put pressure against the joint of the great toe and the first metatarsal and irritate it long before it finally moves the bone out of place.

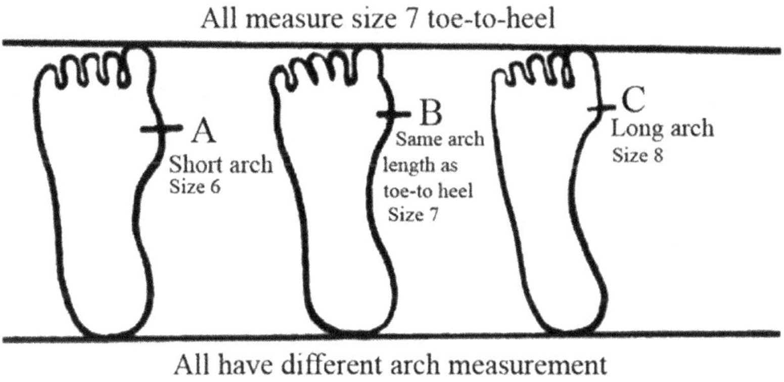

All measure size 7 toe-to-heel

A — Short arch Size 6
B — Same arch length as toe-to heel Size 7
C — Long arch Size 8

All have different arch measurement

Illustration 44

Illustration 44 shows three size 7 feet with three different arch lengths. A is a short arch, B is the same arch size as the toe-to-heel length, and C is a long arch.

The same holds true for the foot with the shorter arch: a size 7 foot with a size six 6 arch measurement, as in illustration 44A, will fall short of the size 7 shoe, putting torque and tension on the great toe joint because the arch isn't long enough for the design of the shoe, and the great toe joint locks from chronic inflammation.

I can use my own feet as an example. My left foot measures a size 6.5 in both the toe-to-heel length and in the arch length. It is perfectly aligned. My right foot measures 6.5 in the toe-to-heel length but with a size 6 arch. The right foot developed a slight bunion.

Had I not started to wear shoes that have no defining arch, the bunion would have worsened. Though my foot is now functional and comfortable most of the time, the damage was done, and I too have to manage inflammation on my right great toe joint whenever I put my foot into a shoe that has a defined arch, such as dress shoes for a wedding.

There are many other foot issues yet to address, but talking about them all would belabor the point, as their onset can be traced to the same origin. Shoes are the culprits of the majority of foot problems and many of the health issues we face.

I hope by now the message is clear. Thirty-five years of practice have given me ample time to study feet, and I can say without a doubt that shoes need to continue to improve in design and function in order for healthy feet to become the norm in our society.

In order for this to happen, a metamorphosis must take place in our mind-set to accept a shoe that is both functional to the foot and aesthetically pleasing.

Fashion can be powerful, provocative, and beautiful, and I look forward to the day when the mentality of the functional shoe becomes fashionable and sexy. I believe we are getting closer to this becoming more of a reality.

(See appendix B for "How to Choose the Right Shoe.")

Conclusion

A cultural change needs to be made regarding our awareness of shoes and the detriment they can be to our health. We did it with the reduction of cigarette smoking, and now it's time for the feet to shine with better health.

Because the feet carry us through space in a very real sense, the feet are the master of our physical reality. Similar to a GPS device, when wearing a shoe that changes the nature of the balanced foot, the brain has to find a new way to redirect and navigate the body to circumvent disaster.

We are born with feet that are perfectly designed to carry us through life's different terrains. The health and function of one's feet will determine how well that individual walks through life, and how efficiently one gets from here to there. Deformities of the feet caused by shoes speak volumes about the constitution of the rest of the body, as evidenced by postural compensation due to weakened feet. Keep in mind posture and emotions are linked, and eventually the macrocosm (the body) will match the microcosm (the feet) and influence one's confidence and mental health.

So why not give the feet as much importance and consideration as we give our hair, face, or teeth? It's a marvel to think of all the productive and powerful energy the feet have to offer the body, and it's astounding to think about how oblivious the average person has become with regard to his or her feet. Choosing shoes without a thought or care as to how it will impact the health of your feet and body seems contrary to all the time and money we invest in keeping the rest of the body healthy.

What is it going to take to accept functional footwear as a normal choice and necessity for overall optimal health and wellness? Women chose to give up girdling their abdomens and hips; now it's time to choose to stop girdling the feet. I'd love to see the day when a commercial is produced mocking the dysfunctional shoe, saying, "I'm sick of this shoe, and I'm not going to wear it anymore!" throwing it out the window in disgust like they did with the bra in the 1970s.

It's time for cobblers to step out of the dark ages and take their rightful place in the shoe industry. Current manufactured shoes are not made well enough to accommodate all the different shapes and sizes of feet.

The earth, a lively and resourceful entity full of abundant nourishment, sustains us physically and can feed us wisdom and connect us to the true essence of our being. It can nurture the seed of potential within us if we allow it. The key to this great connection is to give our feet the freedom to move and feel the grounding benefits the bare or unencumbered foot can receive from the earth. The compassionate brain will be elated and reborn into a newfound, productive, and creative entity because an enormous burden will be lifted from the stress of trying to maneuver the body in a shoe that doesn't fit.

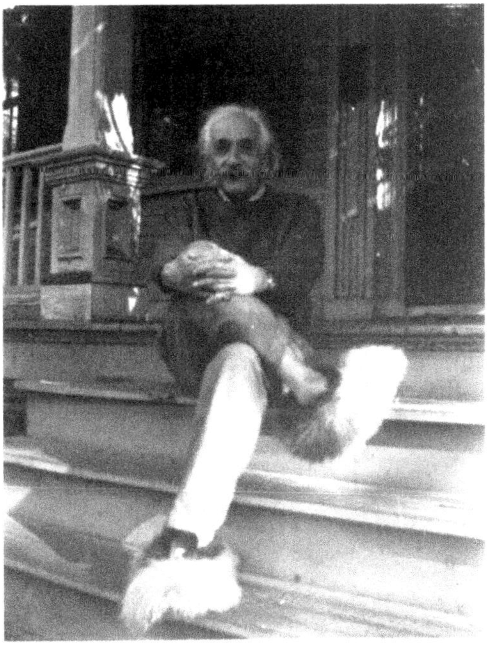

Photo 8

"Einstein in fuzzy slippers." (Gillette, 1905)

Postscript
The Fossils Story

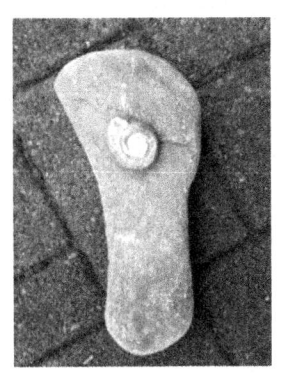

Photo 15

This foot fossil was found on Peaks Island off the coast of Portland, Maine. I found the nautilus fossil while hiking through the Gap of Dunlow in Ireland.

While visiting Peaks Island off the coast of Portland, Maine, my husband and I and some of our nieces and nephews were enjoying time on its very rocky beaches. The stones were huge. The shapes began to speak to us, and we began spontaneously stacking the stones on each other, creating spirited images. It was really exciting and fun, and people walking by stopped and watched and asked, "What do you call this?" as if they had just witnessed a new art form. My husband, barely lifting his head, replied, "Play." I love his simplicity, and on this day it seemed that we were living entities born from the sand of that beach giving life to the past by expressing form out of stones.

Before we left the beach, I felt an intense need to find a heart-shaped stone, which is par for the course with every special trip we take as a memento. That heart shape is symbolic of my love of the experience I had.

Together we combed the beach and the stone piles and did not find a heart-shaped stone, or at least not the one that clearly spoke to me. Neil handed me a stone and said, "This one looks like the shape of a foot." I was slightly interested as he handed it to me, but I continued my search for the heart rock without success.

When we arrived home, I unloaded my luggage and bags and the shells and trinkets I had found and looked at the stone my husband handed to me. I placed it on the floor, and my eyes widened when the stone revealed a true likeness of a foot fossil. Instinctively, as if I were Cinderella trying on the glass slipper, I placed my foot on top of the fossil, and to my amazement my foot and the surface of this beautiful stone fit like a glove. It looked like a cast of the shape and size of my own foot!

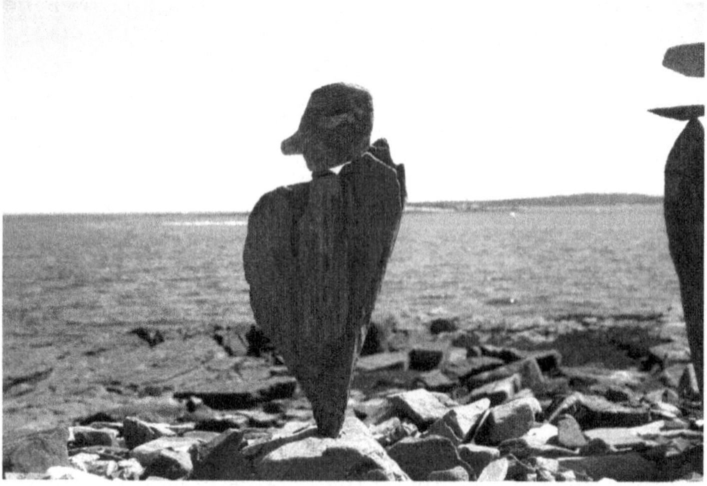

Photo 16

One of the spirited stone images we made on the beach at Peaks Island off the coast of Portland, Maine, which stands about five feet.

Appendix A

Images of Feet in Shoes

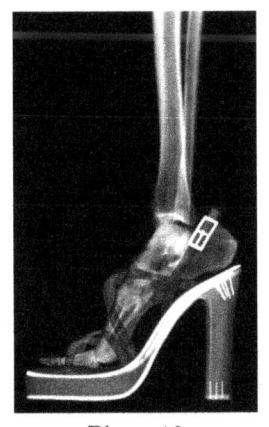

Photo 10

Photo 10 is an x-ray of the lateral view of the right foot and leg as it looks in a high heel.

In photo 10 the angle of the heel bone will encourage inequities in the relationship of the propelling and the balancing muscles of the foot, throwing the foot off its normal mechanics.

See how this shoe directs the foot downward? The toes aren't designed to take the brunt of weight in this position. Observe the hyperextension of these toes even before weight impacts them in this position.

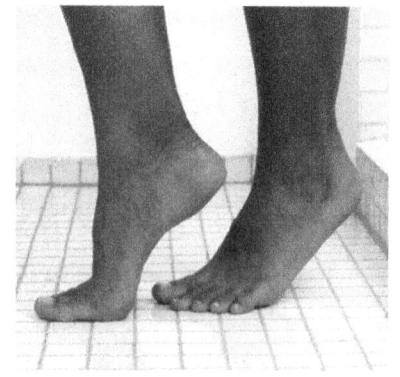

Photo 11

Does the position of the right foot seem like a normal way to walk? For most heel-wearers this mentality is acceptable. It wouldn't be, however, if they understood the consequences and damaging effects.

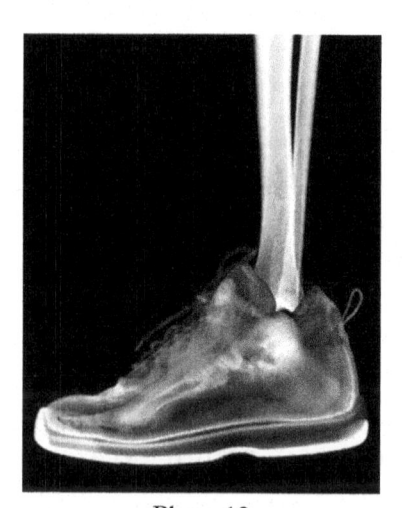

Photo 12

Photo 12 is an x-ray of a healthy position for the foot and body.

Appendix B

How to Choose the Right Shoe

- The following three measurements need to be made by a qualified foot-measurer:
  - 1. Toe-to-heel
  - 2. Ball-to-heel
  - 3. Width
- When getting your feet measured, stand up straight, look forward, and put your full weight on the foot being measured. (Looking down or sitting can change the measurement significantly.)
- After both feet have been measured, choose the longer size even if the other foot is smaller. If the ball-to-heel measurement is longer than the toe-to-heel measurement, you need to choose the ball-to-heel size, and vice versa regarding the longer toe-to-heel in relationship to the arch size. Keep in mind the difference between shoe sizes is only 3/8 of an inch; however, even 1/16 of an inch will create tension if the shoe is too small.
- Try the shoe on your bigger foot first.
- Your thumb should fit comfortably between the back of the shoe and the heel of the foot.
- Walk around in the store with the shoes on. If you feel the slightest bit of pressure or discomfort, they do not fit. Know these sensations will worsen with time.
- Ideally there should be enough room in the toe box of the shoe to tap a pencil tip between every toe while the foot is in the shoe. Wiggle room for your toes is essential for balance.

- Give up the mentality that your shoes need to be broken in. The opposite is true. Your feet will break down to fit in the shoe, and this is not a good thing. The shoe should feel completely comfortable the moment you put your foot into it. There is no "breaking in" period.
- Make sure the shoe fits the shape of your foot. Have someone trace your foot on a piece of flexible cardboard or paper while you stand straight and tall, cut the tracing out and put it in the shoe you want to purchase to see if it fits in the shoe without any folding.
- The shoe should be flexible and fitted to the foot. The shoe should be able to bend fairly easily.
- When trying on a shoe, kick your foot without holding the shoe on with your toes. If it flies off, it is not a good shoe choice. Your sinuses, low back, and hips will suffer with this shoe.
- Ask yourself, "Can I run fast in this shoe?" If the answer is no, it'll trip you up if you ever have to.
- Sport shoes (i.e., ski boots, soccer, etc.) should be the same size as your street shoe, in my opinion.
- Choose a shoe that ties on the foot and has a back on it to keep the foot secure in the shoe.
- Any slip-on shoe should have a back on the heel and the tongue or top of the shoe should cover the surface of the top of the foot.
- Keep in mind that most women's formal shoes are not very functional and should be worn minimally for the occasion, and not on a regular basis.
    (They have the potential to cause damage in one evening.)
- Flip-flops should be reserved for the beach if ever worn at all. They were originally intended as protective wear from the hot sand on the beach and not for distance walking. This innocent little foam rubber thong is one of the worst causes of broken arches (hyper-pronation) and bunions.

I love shoes, and being a bit of a "fashionista," I too want my shoes to match the panache of my dress when I am going to a special event, and I admit this shoe is usually not very functional for the foot. The key here is to wear them sparingly, knowing that this is not an everyday shoe. Understand that there will be repercussions in deciding to wear a shoe that limits foot function on a regular basis, or even for just a walk around the block. Invest in function whenever possible.

There are a lot of attractive, functional shoes out there since the shoe market has become more accommodating toward the need for better foot function. So have fun, and happy shoe shopping!

Appendix C

How to Measure Feet using a Brannock Measuring Device

Please note: you will *not* get an accurate measurement if you measure your own feet.

Stand straight with head and eyes looking forward.

Each foot must be resting on the device with the heel all the way to the back, and allow full weight on the foot being measured. The measurements are as follows: (See Photo 14 "Brannock Measuring Device.")

1. Toe-to-heel: measures the vertical length of the foot at its longest. Keep in mind the second toe is often longer than the great toe, so the measurement should be reflected as such.
2. Ball-to-heel: measures the vertical length of the area from the heel to the (metatarsal phalangeal joint) MPJ of the great toe.
3. The width measures the horizontal area at the widest part of the foot (from the ball of the great toe to the ball of the fifth toe).

Measuring the Foot

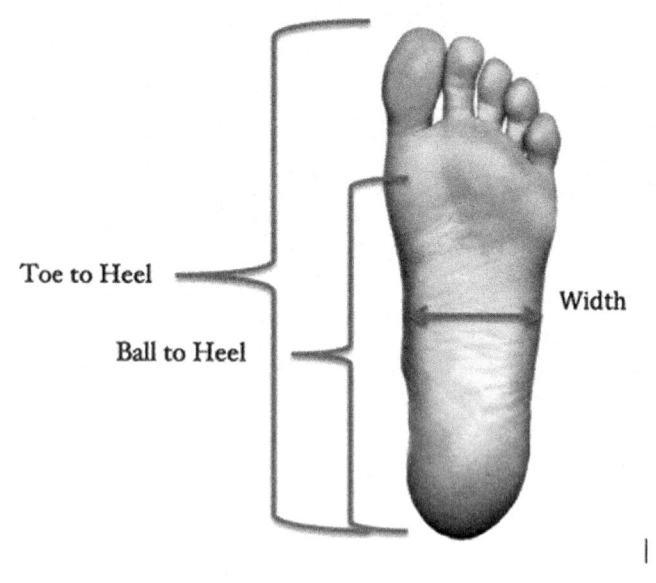

Photo 13

Three necessary foot measurements

- 70 percent of the people have a longer ball-to-heel size
- 10 percent have a shorter ball-to-heel size
- This is why 80 percent have foot problems

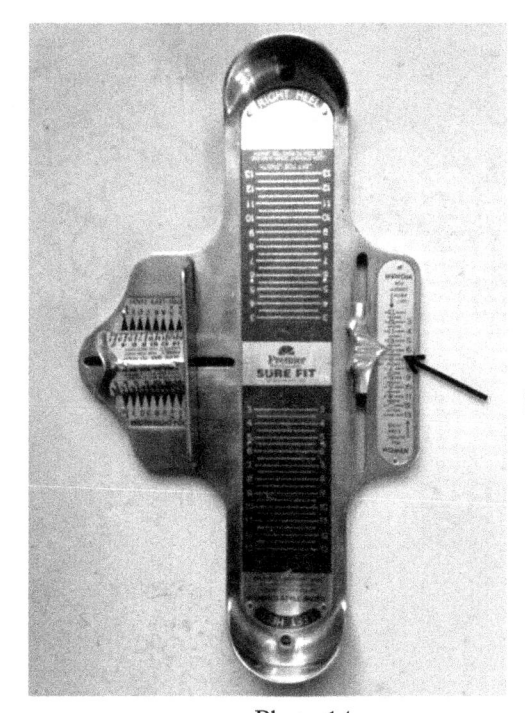

Photo 14

Brannock Measuring Device

The arch of the foot is measured with the knob along the side of the device, which is designed for the placement of the ball of the foot.

Appendix D

Walking and the body as a microcosm interact like this:

Illustration 45

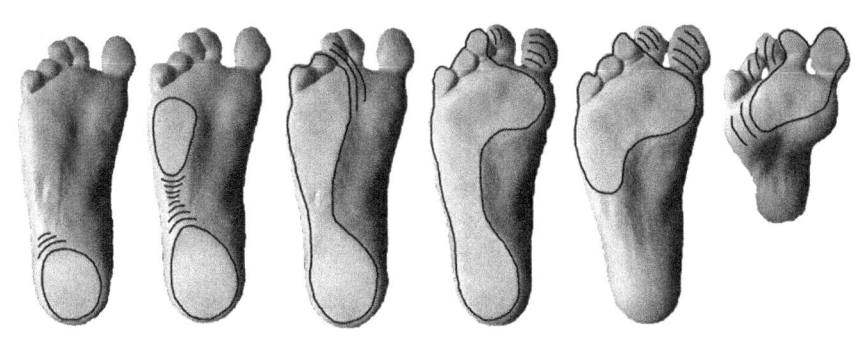

Illustration 45 shows the distribution of weight on the foot in one step walking barefoot.

This is the process:

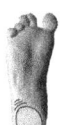

A. When the foot lifts from the floor, the pelvis tilts under. When the heel contacts the floor, it engages the pelvis and the muscles along the upper lateral leg become activated.

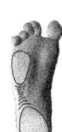

B. The pivotal movement of the talus initiates the movement of the ball and socket of the hip joint with the same degree and directs weight along the lateral column of the foot to the cuboid, which is the "keystone" of foot movement. The muscles connecting the hip to the knee then contract and the leg becomes mobile.

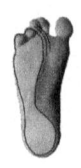

C. Articulation of the cuboid and fourth and fifth metatarsal joints engages the transverse arch to carry the momentum of movement from supination of the lateral column to gently pronate the foot toward the medial column. The ball and sockets of the shoulder and jaw joints glide with this movement.

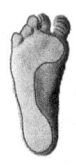

D. The flexible and capable arch of the foot absorbs the weight of the body, which initiates movement of the spine, allowing the curves of the back to receive the wave and sway into propelling motion. This creates efficient communication of neural signals to the glands, organs, and muscles.

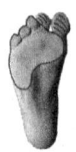

E. As weight reaches the ball of the foot, the upper back and chest receive a cushion of impact, provided by the toe extensors and interosseous muscles between the metatarsals, to keep vitality and momentum moving up toward the neck and head.

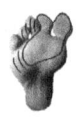

F. The action of the great toe and small toe flexor muscles engage the metatarsal and phalangeal joints to bend, providing tremendous strength to stabilize the chest, neck, and head during the last process of this step in movement.

The articulation and strength of the fourth and fifth phalanges (toes) will determine the structural ability to keep the shoulders, neck, and head stable and in the line of gravity in the process of movement.

The strength of toes 1, 2, and 3 will determine the elasticity and flow of movement of the cervical vertebrae. Each toe shares equal weight before the spring muscles of the great toe and arch thrust the foot off the ground.

Appendix E

Dr. Hiss' Seven Fundamental Functions of the Foot (1933)

- *Support:* The ability to withstand weight.

- *Balance:* Control of body weight over the center of gravity.

- *Locomotion:* Coordination of muscles to move joints for propelling the body through space.

- *Adaptability:* Coordination of support, balance, and locomotion to compensate for changed position.

- *Distribution:* Control of contact pressure made by the sole of the foot on the ground with momentum.

- *Vitality:* Life that manifests itself in the feet as well as the rest of the body. Vitality is the body's innate intelligence and its ability to maintain the essence of living.

- *Power:* Refers to the action of the muscles that transform chemical energy into mechanical energy.

Works Cited

Amazing facts about the human body, health and the intelligence within us all... (n.d.). Retrieved July 12, 2016, from http://www.cafeoflifepikespeak.com/amazing_facts.htm

FitzGerald, W.H., Dr., Bower, E. F., Dr. *Zone Therapy*. Columbus, Ohio: I. W Long, 1917.

From Louis XIV to Christian Louboutin: A History of Red-Soled Shoes. (2016). Retrieved July 08, 2016, from http://www.forbes.com/pictures/emjl45ghf/louis-xiv-of-france-posing-in-red-heeled-shoes/#7b26eb5e1893

Gillette G., Einstein in Fuzzy Slippers Princeton University, Princeton, New Jersey: In D. D. McCormack (Comp.), 1905.

Hiss, J. M., Dr. *New Feet for Old*. Garden City, New York: Doubleday, Doran & Company, Inc., 1933.

Hiss, J. M., Dr. *Functional foot disorders* (3rd ed.). Los Angeles, CA: Oxford Press, 1949.

Hoffman, P., Dr. *Conclusions Drawn from a Comparative Study of the Feet of Barefooted and Shoe-wearing Peoples*. Volume III, Number 2: *The American Journal of Orthopedic Surgery*, 1905.

Issel, Christine, *Reflexology: Art, Science & History*, Sacramento, CA: New Frontier Publishing, 2014.

Myers, T. (n.d.). Anatomy Trains. Retrieved July 16, 2016, from http://www.optp.com/Anatomy-Trains

Silverstein, A. *Human Anatomy & Physiology.* United States: Wiley & Sons, Inc., 1980.

Sadler, T.W., & Langman, J. *Langman's Medical Embryology.* 8th Edition. Philadelphia: Lippincott William & Wilkins, 2010.

Shakespeare, W., & McEachern, C. *The Life and Death of King John.* New York, NY: Penguin Books, 2000.

Shoes in the 1800s. (n.d.). Retrieved July 12, 2016, from http://people.seas.harvard.edu/~jones/mckay/history.html

Think About It Thursday: How Far Does The Average Human Walk In A Lifetime? (2015, July 30). Retrieved July 12, 2016, from https://sciencemadefun.net/blog/think-about-it-thursday-how-far-does-the-average-human-walk-in-a-lifetime/

Thinkstock by Getty Images. Purchase date: 11.22.2014, Purchase #: 14001161

Tuchscherer, M., Dr. (1993). *An Introduction to Peripheral and Central Reflex Activity: A Means of Understanding Reflexology.*

Wikler, S.J. *Your Feet are Killing You.* New York: Fell, 1953.

Wikler, S.J. *Take Off Your Shoes and Walk: Steps to Better Foot Health.* New York: Devin-Adair, 1961.

Index

A

accessory 75, 92
Achilles tendon 31, 90, 92, 94, 108, 122
Adaptability 149
adaptable 28, 73
ankle 29, 60, 62, 81, 82, 91, 96, 105
anterior 82, 101, 103, 106
arch 13, 14, 18, 25, 26, 27, 44, 45, 52, 64, 68, 69, 70, 71, 73, 74, 75, 83, 84, 91, 92, 94, 95, 96, 97, 98, 99, 100, 101, 102, 103, 104, 113, 114, 115, 116, 117, 122, 123, 127, 128, 129, 139, 145, 148
arch supports 69, 98, 113, 115, 116
arteries 108
arthritis 122
articulation 22, 23, 81, 148
attachment 31, 43, 89, 91, 93, 94, 95, 96, 100, 101, 102, 120, 121, 123
avulsion 96, 102, 121

B

babies 76
balance xviii, 12, 14, 18, 19, 23, 27, 30, 31, 34, 42, 43, 48, 49, 52, 53, 63, 68, 73, 76, 81, 90, 92, 97, 100, 109, 120, 122, 139, 149
ball-to-heel 139, 143, 144
barefoot xvii, xviii, 9, 54, 71, 76, 77, 82, 87, 116, 147

bladder 98
blisters 119, 127
blood xix, 1, 3, 14, 18, 23, 26, 34, 53, 55, 63, 69, 94, 108, 109, 110, 111, 122
bone spur 120, 121
brain 10, 21, 22, 23, 26, 34, 35, 36, 39, 41, 53, 69, 75, 76, 131, 132
bunion 58, 60, 70, 100, 126, 127, 128, 129

C

calcaneus 62, 78, 81, 91, 122
calluses 58, 59, 60, 119, 127
cancer 43, 48, 86
cartilage 74, 76
cervical 23, 106, 148
children xviii, 3, 4, 75, 77, 85
chronic strain 58, 104, 106
collapse 69, 71, 104
compensation xiv, xv, 18, 19, 23, 26, 28, 40, 42, 43, 48, 54, 63, 77, 90, 102, 109, 110, 131
congestion 53, 54
constipation 3, 102
corns 119, 127
correction vii, ix, 75, 115, 126
cramps 119
cuboid 62, 64, 69, 70, 74, 92, 101, 122, 124, 125, 126, 147, 148
cuneiform 99

D

deform 74, 85
deformity 13, 71, 78, 90, 96
degenerative 14, 22, 24, 28, 53, 86, 108
deoxygenated 63, 109
digits 62
dislocation 58, 60, 70, 71
disorder xv, 43
distribution xv, 42, 53, 81, 147, 149
Dr. Hiss ix, 13, 14, 30, 73, 74, 121, 149
Dr. Hoffman 83, 84, 85, 86
Dr. Wikler ix, 14, 22, 48, 77, 86, 107, 110, 111

E

elimination 48, 109
exercise 54, 97, 115
exhaustion 59, 63, 89
extension 62, 105, 109
extensor hallucis 105

F

fascia 89, 90, 92, 104, 120
fatigue 64, 65, 89, 100, 103, 104, 108
femoral triangle 110
fibula 81, 99
flat feet 74
flexible 14, 15, 55, 62, 77, 115, 140, 148
flexion 62
flip flop 123
foot measure 129
function vii, ix, xv, xviii, 3, 10, 12, 14, 15, 18, 19, 23, 26, 27, 28, 30, 40, 42, 43, 48, 49, 53, 59, 62, 64, 65, 68, 69, 70, 71, 74, 77, 81, 87, 92, 94, 96, 97, 98, 102, 104, 108, 113, 114, 116, 125, 130, 131, 141

G

gait 62, 107, 127
gastrocnemius 31, 90, 91, 108, 120
glands 18, 26, 148
gravitational line 29, 30, 63
groin 106, 110

H

hallux rigidous 106
hamstring 94, 109
head 4, 15, 22, 23, 35, 38, 39, 42, 48, 53, 68, 99, 100, 135, 143, 148
health vii, ix, xi, 1, 5, 6, 8, 14, 18, 34, 39, 43, 49, 54, 81, 86, 95, 107, 108, 113, 114, 115, 116, 130, 131, 132, 151, 152
heart xix, 22, 31, 94, 107, 108, 109, 111, 136
heel 10, 13, 27, 30, 31, 39, 48, 52, 53, 60, 62, 65, 77, 78, 90, 91, 92, 94, 108, 109, 120, 121, 122, 128, 129, 137, 138, 139, 140, 143, 144, 147
heel spur 120
hinge 60, 81, 91
hip 12, 29, 64, 98, 101, 102, 108, 110, 119, 147, 148
hyper-pronate 75, 104

I

iliopsoas 106
immobilize 69
inflammatory 42, 105, 106
intermediate 92
intestinal 101, 102

J

jaw 106, 119, 148
joints 12, 19, 23, 28, 44, 59, 62, 64, 75, 81, 82, 92, 124, 148, 149

K

knee 12, 27, 29, 64, 81, 89, 90, 94, 97, 100, 101, 109, 119, 148

L

lactic acid 63
lateral 18, 52, 58, 62, 64, 65, 69, 74, 92, 98, 101, 124, 125, 137, 147, 148
lateral column 62, 64, 65, 147, 148
life 6, 7, 8, 31, 38, 39, 58, 59, 60, 74, 78, 81, 87, 117, 125, 131, 135, 149, 152
ligaments 12, 40, 42, 43, 48, 59, 60, 65, 71, 73, 81, 83, 91, 92, 101, 104, 105, 114, 122
locomotion 26, 64, 68, 81, 98, 149
long foot muscles 12, 31, 89, 90, 95
longitudinal arch 74, 83, 84
low back 27, 44, 94, 98, 104, 114, 119, 140
lower leg xiv, 30, 43, 52, 59, 60, 81, 89, 95, 97, 99, 105, 108, 122
lumbar 106
lymph 26, 53, 55, 109

M

medial 18, 45, 52, 62, 64, 74, 75, 92, 99, 124, 125, 148
medial column 62, 64, 75, 148
misalignment 18, 42, 59, 64, 75, 98, 106, 114, 127
momentum 52, 69, 148, 149
Morton's neuroma 71, 123, 125
movement xvii, 12, 14, 18, 23, 26, 27, 30, 31, 42, 43, 44, 52, 53, 54, 62, 63, 64, 69, 70, 71, 74, 75, 77, 81, 83, 89, 90, 101, 103, 104, 108, 114, 115, 127, 147, 148

N

navicular 62, 74, 75
neck 23, 27, 34, 48, 53, 58, 59, 68, 106, 114, 119, 148
nerve xv, 18, 23, 35, 39, 113, 123, 124, 125
nervous system xiii, xv, 18, 26, 36, 39, 40, 55, 122

O

organ xii, xiii, 18, 34, 75, 109

P

pancreas 104
pelvis 27, 106, 109, 123, 147
phalanges 62, 148
plantar fasciitis 71, 92, 122
PNF 60
posterior tibialis 97, 98, 103
posture 26, 30, 31, 40, 43, 48, 63, 77, 82, 84, 109, 131
power xviii, 26, 31, 46, 49, 51, 52, 70, 73, 81, 89, 116, 123, 127, 149
pressure 1, 13, 14, 21, 34, 38, 39, 68, 71, 85, 93, 108, 120, 128, 139, 149
pronation 69, 101, 140
propel 31, 53, 110
props vii, 73, 97, 104, 113, 114, 116
prostate 98
protect 71, 77, 92, 93, 104
pump bump 92, 94
purpose 7, 8, 11, 19, 90, 104

R

reflex xii, 3, 4, 16, 21, 22, 33, 34, 35, 42, 43, 44, 89, 95, 97, 99, 102, 103, 105, 152
reflexology, reflexing x, xi, xii, xiii, xiv, xv, 2, 3, 4, 5, 6, 7, 8, 14, 15, 16,

18, 19, 22, 23, 24, 35, 38, 39, 40, 41, 42, 43, 44, 45, 55, 57, 60, 122
reflex sites 21, 42, 43, 89, 95, 97, 99, 105
rehabilitation 74, 111, 116
retinacula 105
rigid 14, 15, 26, 39, 53, 54, 58, 59, 69, 70, 94, 97, 114, 116
runner 94

S

sciatica 102
sesamoid 77, 81, 92, 93
shin splints 103, 104
shock absorb 70, 94, 104
shoes xi, xvii, xviii, 1, 9, 10, 11, 12, 13, 14, 22, 23, 26, 28, 31, 40, 42, 48, 54, 55, 58, 59, 62, 65, 68, 69, 70, 73, 76, 77, 78, 85, 86, 87, 89, 91, 94, 95, 96, 97, 98, 99, 100, 102, 105, 106, 107, 108, 111, 115, 116, 117, 119, 120, 123, 125, 127, 128, 129, 130, 131, 132, 137, 139, 140, 141, 151, 152
shoe-wearing 82, 83, 85, 151
soleus 31, 90, 108, 120
spine 18, 23, 25, 26, 30, 35, 44, 63, 106, 113, 114, 115, 148
sprain 96, 102
spring 18, 52, 62, 64, 69, 70, 71, 74, 94, 98, 106, 114, 148
stable 30, 64, 65, 68, 69, 96, 148
stomach 104
Structural Reflexology x
supinate 69, 71
supination 65, 69, 96, 148
support x, 53, 68, 70, 107, 114, 149
surgery ix, 38, 44, 58, 82, 83, 84, 85, 86, 122, 125, 126, 151

syndrome 120, 124

T

talus 60, 62, 78, 81, 91, 114, 122, 123, 147
tendonitis 71
tension xiv, xv, xviii, xix, 12, 15, 19, 23, 26, 28, 30, 39, 40, 42, 43, 55, 58, 59, 60, 65, 90, 92, 94, 96, 99, 100, 101, 102, 103, 106, 108, 115, 116, 120, 121, 122, 127, 129, 139
theories 37
thoracic 58
throat 106
thyroid 58, 101, 106
tibia 81, 123
toe-to-heel 13, 128, 129, 139, 143
transverse arch 64, 69, 70, 71, 91, 92, 101, 104, 114, 127, 148
trauma 7, 34, 73, 89, 115, 122

U

uterus 48, 98

V

varicosities 94
veins 108, 109
vertebra 26, 148
vitality xi, xviii, 14, 34, 39, 40, 54, 87, 98, 115, 116, 117, 125, 127, 148, 149

W

weight bearing 51, 64, 70, 75, 83
wellness 46, 132

X

x-ray 75, 78, 122, 125, 137, 138